D1622223

PRACTICE
OF GERIATRIC
PSYCHIATRY

PRACTICE
OF GERIATRIC
PSYCHIATRY

Alex Comfort

ELSEVIER • NEW YORK
New York • Oxford

Elsevier North Holland, Inc.
52 Vanderbilt Avenue, New York, New York 10017

Distributors outside the United States and Canada:

Thomond Books
(A Division of Elsevier/North-Holland Scientific Publishers, Ltd.)
P.O. Box 85
Limerick, Ireland

Library of Congress Cataloging in Publication Data

Comfort, Alexander, 1920–
    Practice of geriatric psychiatry.

    Bibliography: p.
    Includes index.
    1. Geriatric psychiatry. I. Title.
    [DNLM: 1. Geriatric psychiatry. WT150 C732p]
RC451.4.A5C63   618.9′76′89   79-24444
ISBN 0-444-00360-6

Desk Editor   Gail Huggins
Design   Edmée Froment
Production Manager   Joanne Jay
Compositor   Lexigraphics, Inc.
Printer   Haddon Craftsmen

Manufactured in the United States of America

CONTENTS

PREFACE

The medical care of older patients will account for an increasing proportion of the daily work of every physician now in practice or in training, other than those who intend to limit their work to pediatrics or obstetrics. This will be true in every specialism, but particularly in primary care or family practice—the medical discipline which best delivers geriatric care, and which, in countries with developed geriatric medicine, is the chief means of providing it.

This book presents "geriatric psychiatry" not as a specialty, but as something which forms a part of the professional equipment with which every doctor works. The primary care physician, the internist, and the surgeon all see and need to recognize mental health problems. There is a special need for physicians to be skilled in handling these problems in older patients, because however much physical and mental health interact in the young, in the older patient, they are wholly inseparable for practical and clinical purposes. Mental confusion may be the sole presenting symptom of physical illness or overmedication, but most patients with classically "mental" problems will also have physical problems, and the social repercussions of age expressed in the attitudes of society, of the patient, and of the doctor have profound effects on the outcome of physical illness and physical treatment.

Expertise in this area is now accordingly a professional necessity. A necessary mark of good geriatric practice is that the doctor who first sees the elderly patient should possess that expertise. Like pediatrics, geriatrics is a distinct body of clinical skills, but it is also an attitude of mind—one which runs, in many respects, counter to cultural indoctrination and to what one learns in medical school. One major reason to address the study of geriatric psychiatry lies in its effect on doctors themselves, on their capacity to examine their attitudes toward aging in themselves and others, and consequently on their

entire practice of medicine with this particular age group. The wholly erroneous notions that "the old" are untreatable, and for biological reasons not
worth treating, that infirmity in later life can be explained by chronology
alone, and that what cannot be cured is best addressed by sympathy and
benign neglect have been signally exploded in European medical education
by the growth of a vigorous, curative, and supportive geriatric medicine which
produces results. Old people in America are entitled to the same degree of
medical re-education in those whom they consult, and they are about to
demand it. Readiness to meet this demand is both necessary to the doctor's
self-esteem and immensely rewarding in practice.

I have tried to organize the content of this book in the way which can best
give practical help in achieving this readiness to colleagues in the widest range
of fields. My own experience in America has been idiosyncratic, in that I have
worked in a geriatric psychiatry unit which received consultation cases, and
hence those in whom a "psychiatric" diagnosis had been made after physical
factors had been eliminated, but it is possible, even in these cases, to appreciate how they presented to the physician who first saw them. The first
chapter is an overview of the subject; the second deals with the diagnosis of
"senility", which is not in itself a diagnosis so much as a signal to investigate
and make a diagnosis.

These two introductory chapters can be read by themselves; their content is
treated in more detail in the subsequent chapters. They deal with the clinical
aspects of psychosis, dementia, clinical testing, psychotherapy, special problems such as bereavement and sleeplessness in the old, and the pattern of
organization for health care delivery. These are the areas in which we might
wish our advisers to have skills when we ourselves require health care in age.
Even for those to whom this prospect is now remote, it provides a salutary
focus of identification with patients who are there now.

A book on geriatric psychiatry necessarily deals both with drugs and with
the "nonmedicalized model." Old people are the victims both of real losses
and of cultural rejection. When mentally ill, they also represent—because
they have lived with their earlier problems into old age—a retrospective
critique of our skills in treating mental illness and, indeed, of our psychiatry
in general.

The nonpsychiatrist doctor needs to remember—since it is rarely taught in
this form in psychiatry courses—that what is now called "psychiatry" is a
double medical enterprise, involving two quite different tasks, and geriatric
psychiatry is no exception. One task is that of assisting typically reacting
humans in handling typical human experiences (often referred to as "counseling"). The other is that of assisting patients whose experience is ab initio
atypical in quality by reason of the way in which they perceive it, or perceive
and mobilize their reactions to it. The distinction was obvious to the old
physician—alienist. It became somewhat obscured as psychodynamics, developmental psychiatry, and psychoanalysis indicated the structure and content of such atypical responses, but the distinction is again becoming clear and

will become still more evident with the practical application of neuropharmacology. With psychotics, this is an easy enough idea to grasp, but the group of "neurotics," meaning those who have learned unprofitable reactions early, includes many who have never had the consistent experience of firing reliably on all six mental cylinders. Classical psychiatry has had little to say about individual durability, beyond noting that all equations between childhood experience and later pathology fail to predict who will respond by illness to a relatively ordinary childhood and who will survive a horrendous one intact. In this process, failure to give developmental passwords and low resilience—a better-defined version of what used to be labeled "psychasthenia"—certainly bend the twig. Learning to manipulate the perceived world in terms of the patient's perceived limitations then takes over.

Geriatric psychiatry is confronted with the end result, plus any new losses. Discursive psychotherapy can obviously support both groups, and psychoanalytic psychotherapy, through which both typical and atypical experiences acquire some kind of structure, can be educative. The lifelong malfunctions for whom our limited armamentarium happens to provide a replacement part is, however, the real test of our therapeutics—the "neurotic" or "borderline patient" for whom nominal doses of lithium, an antipsychotic, a tricyclic, or even thyroid hormone supplementation reconnects a loose ignition lead, to use a mechanical analogy, and restores normal response to the throttle. These clear-cut cases are at present relatively exceptional, either because our therapeutics are still crude or because a deficit in childhood may have been self-curing and have left scars in the form of functionally autonomous learned reactions. Discursive psychotherapists who eschew medication and "lay" psychotherapists who do not know any medicine never see these cases for reasons of observer bias. Since intervention is never too late, given ongoing malfunction, and since one major mission of geriatrics is the rescue of the misdiagnosed, the geriatrician should be alert for them. These patients will indeed need psychotherapy as well as medication, but with the difference that they will now be able to profit from it, and for this nobody is too old if the intervention is well placed. The competent doctor will eschew neither psychotherapy nor medication; treating either as a closed system implies only lack of clinical judgment. He will neither medicalize grief, social injustice, poverty, and loss by treating them with sedatives, nor try to counsel a faulty ignition system back into function (though if he cannot reconnect the faulty lead, he may have to counsel his patient on coaxing better function out of the deficient system). The crudity of this analogy is deliberate. Discursive psychiatry inflates the physician and goes to the head of the student; indiscriminate medication saves office time and protects the physician against having to use judgment or acquire self-knowledge. Sensible eclecticism is harder work, but it produces better patient care.

CREDITS FOR
TABLES AND FIGURE

The author thanks the following publishers and authors for permission to reproduce published tabular or pictorial materials:

TABLE 3.1. Modified from Lippmann, S. Depression—A good approach for the non-psychiatrist. III—How to use the tricyclics. Resident and Staff Physician, August 1978, 111–117. Reprinted by permission of Romaine Pierson, Port Washington, New York.

TABLE 3.2. Freedman R. and Schwab, P.J. Paranoid symptoms in patients on a general hospital psychiatric unit. Archives of General Psychiatry 35:387–390. Copyright 1978, American Medical Association. Reprinted by permission.

TABLE 3.3. Adapted from Manschreck, T. The assessment of paranoid features. Comprehensive Psychiatry 20:370–377, 1979. Reprinted by permission of Grune & Stratton, Inc., New York. Symptoms were described in a previous article: Manschreck, T. and Petri, M. The paranoid syndrome. Lancet ii:251–253, 1978.

TABLES 4.1–4.3. Marsden, C.D. The diagnosis of dementia. In Isaacs, A.D. and Post, F. (eds) Studies in Geriatric Psychiatry, 1978. Reprinted by permission of John Wiley & Sons Ltd, Chichester.

TABLES 4.4 and 4.5. Seltzer, B. and Sherwin, I. Organic brain syndrome: An empirical study and critical review. The American Journal of Psychiatry, Vol. 134, pp. 16–21, 1978. Copyright 1978, the American Psychiatric Association. Reprinted by permission.

TABLE 4.6. Hachinski, V.C. et al. Multi-infarct dementia. A cause of mental deterioration in the elderly. Lancet ii:207–210, 1974. Reprinted by permission of Lancet Ltd.

TABLE 4.7. Yesavage, J.A. et al. Vasodilators in senile dementias. Archives of General Psychiatry 36:220–223, 1979. Copyright 1979, American Medical Association. Reprinted by permission.

TABLE 8.1. Strouthidis, T.M. Medical requirements of a day hospital. Gerontologia Clinica 16:241–247, 1974. Reprinted by permission of S. Karger AG, Basel.

FIGURE 8.1. Hall, M.R.P. *In* Irvine, R.E. (ed) Symposium on day care. Gerontologia Clinica, Vol. 16, Nos. 5 and 6, 1974. Reprinted by permission of S. Karger AG, Basel.

PRACTICE
OF GERIATRIC
PSYCHIATRY

1
INTRODUCTION
AND OVERVIEW

It is to the physician, not the psychiatrist, that the old and their relatives turn for crisis intervention. This is fitting, for at no period of life are mental and physical symptoms more closely interlinked. The physician who treats old patients must either address their mental problems, at least by understanding their relation to nonpsychiatric medication, or run the risk of being actively pathogenic. It is, moreover, the physician who, by careful physical examination, can save the old from psychiatric institutional commitment and restore them to worthwhile living, an immensely satisfying exercise when it works. So much geriatric psychiatry, then, is part of the normal equipment of all who see patients over the age of 65.

Old people suffer from the psychiatric problems common to the human condition. They also suffer from psychiatric problems peculiar to age, and peculiar to age in our culture. Peculiar to age is the tendency for physical diseases which earlier in life present sharply and specifically to present in geriatric practice in a muted or nonspecific form. Typical syndromes are blurred: Coronary heart disease, pneumonia, urinary infection, thyrotoxicosis, and many other medical conditions may be stripped of their usual signatures and appear as a nonspecific combination of mental and physical symptoms such as withdrawal, mental blunting, loss of mobility, and physical weakness. This syndrome, popularly called "senility," represents the Shakespearian "last act." So far from being a diagnosis, senility is the geriatric equivalent of failure to thrive in infants (Hodkinson, 1976). Moreover, mental failure may be the sole presenting symptom of a wide range of pathologies in the old, many of them remediable and some of them iatrogenic. Of all old people who present with a "psychiatric" problem, between 10 and 30%, according to age, owe their illness to an undiagnosed medical condition, or to the effects of medication, or to both. The older the patient, the more often are psychiatric disorders symptomatic, and the first stop must be with the geriatric physician.

THE CLIENTELE OF "GERIATRIC PSYCHIATRY"

Cases referred to a geriatric psychiatry unit include three types of patients: those with missed symptomatic mental impairment due to identifiable illness or drugs, those with newly appearing dementia or psychosis requiring expert consultation and diagnosis, and those with some psychiatric feature who are otherwise uninteresting to the general physician and can, by reason of age, be unloaded on a geriatric unit.

Prevalence of the first type of case will depend on the standard of geriatric diagnosis in primary care—they are more common in America than in Britain but occur in both countries. Cases of the second kind are clearly proper referrals. Cases of the third kind include the longstanding Parkinsonian patient who develops dementia or hallucinations, either from the disease or as a side effect, and the patient with residual cerebral damage from any cause who wanders, is aggressive, or otherwise resists disposal. This material, although unpromising in the eyes of those who refer the patients, is an important area for research. A geriatric unit can develop the expertise in medication needed to make life as bearable as possible for those who reach old age irremediably sick, and for their relatives.

More than at any other age, however, "senile" patients who do not respond to an exclusionary search for simple causes illustrate the confluence of pathology, age, and life situation. A typical example is the subject with longstanding personality problems who has had a stroke and shows intellectual impairment, who has suffered the loss of a spouse, who can no longer cope with his family situation, whose money has run out, and whose life-support systems have collapsed. Disease, the backlog of problems previously in equilibrium, bereavement, the social devaluation of the old in our culture, and poverty tend to strike together. Physician, psychiatrist, neuropharmacologist, and social worker may not "cure" these ills, although they can alleviate and, sometimes, heal. If such a collusion of misfortune occurred in younger adults, it would be a focus of sympathy and of intensive research. Good geriatrics and better social attitudes may bring similar support to the old.

THE CULTURAL PROBLEM: GERONTOPHOBIA

Unique to our culture is its rejection of the old, their exclusion from work and their accustomed social space, their premature burial by society as "un-people," and a rich and erroneous folklore of mental decline, infirmity, asexuality, ineducability, and the normality of causeless mental disorder in the old. Because this folklore is shared both by the old themselves and, unfortunately, by physicians, mental ill health as well as physical is seen as requiring no explanation, provided the subject is "old." At the same time, the rejecting attitude of society, and fear of being judged senile, forms a ground-bass to every theme of mental illness in old age and must constantly be addressed by a corrective psychotherapy designed to restore self-esteem. Often this need be no more than contact with a physician who does not project dislike or contempt for old people.

Geriatric psychiatry is best introduced to students—who need prophylactic injections against the notion that aging involves imbecility, that geriatric medicine is a branch of embalming, and that geropsychiatry is uninteresting and useless—by a series of aphorisms. The first is that older people are responsive to treatment. Not only are many apparent psychiatric disorders symptomatic, but also, if psychiatric disorders are treatable in the young, they are treatable in the old, and the same methods are appropriate. The second is that old people are not normally sick or crazy: Seventy-five percent of those over 65 describe themselves as "well," and Jacques Cousteau diving in his 70s or Artur Rubinstein performing at 90 are more representative of "normal" age than a sufferer from organic brain disease. Old people who "become crazy" do so because they always have been crazy, because they are sick, or because we drive them crazy. Major primary psychosis rarely makes its first unheralded appearance in old age: Depression may do so, but florid schizoprenia virtually never, if we except the "late paraphrenia" occurring in patients with a lifetime of odd beliefs, which responds extremely well to antipsychotic drugs. As for sickness, it is characteristic of age that disorientation and confusion are relatively easily induced by infection, toxicity, electrolyte changes, and other physical causes, as are convulsions in infants. Social ostracism apart, the most common cause of sudden, unexplained mental illness in the old is medication—self-administered, doctor administered, or borrowed from neighbors. Accordingly, the first psychodiagnostic step is the withdrawal of all medication which is not life sustaining and the review of medication which is. The "plastic bag test"—provision of a plastic bag in which all medication without exception is to be placed—may yield dozens or even scores of preparations. As a corollary, the student must be aware that in view of the increased homeostatic instability of age, the prescription of any drug in old age is no light matter. For the old, there is no such thing as a minor tranquilizer. Neurological and biochemical reserves are reduced, multiple pathology may be present, iatrogenic disease of all kinds, especially psychiatric, can be precipitated by modest doses of many agents, and falls caused by hypotension, ataxia, or confusion can cause the patient's death.

Finally, chronic brain syndrome is neither an inevitable concomitant of age, if one lives long enough, nor is it the commonest major psychiatric disorder.

The most common psychiatric disorder in age is depression. Not only is age in our culture depressing, but there is a basic neuroendocrine shift with aging in the direction characteristic of affective disorder (Finch, 1976). Depression may be reactive or endogenous, it can be agitated and suicidal, but quite commonly, and more commonly than in the young, it can be confined to somatic equivalents—backache, fatigue, cancer phobia. It can also present as pseudodementia or confusion, or as anhedonia, including loss of libido.

Depression in the old is commonly undiagnosed. It is the most likely underlying basis for unexplained sudden or gradual downhill change once sickness and medication are excluded, and it is a medical emergency, both because of the high risk of suicide or death from "giving up," and because it is treatable, often with spectacular benefit. Even when some underlying brain damage exists, lightening of depression can restore social function. When an old person withdraws into self-neglect and isolation, this is far more commonly the result of endogenous depression than the cause of reactive depression. Bereavement, which increases in frequency with age to include friends and peers as well as spouses, and skills or achievements as well as persons, can determine its onset, although grief and sorrow are not diseases and should not be medicated. Loss (see Chapter 6) is one of the inevitable features of human age, and it cannot be rendered wholly painless.

"Late-life depressions deserve the most serious and even heroic therapeutic efforts, regardless of the age of the patient" (Linn, 1975). Many respond to tricyclic agents, but the dose must initially be reduced, because delirium and acute retention are easily induced in the old. One-third adult maintenance doses of amitryptilene or doxepin are typically effective. The drugs with more marked anticholinergic effects should be used with care. Antidepressant drugs should be given at night in a single bolus in order that side effects may be covered by sleep. Early waking is diagnostic of depression in the old, but the temptation to supplement sedative tricyclics with sedatives should be resisted except on a very short-term basis. In unresponsive depression, neither monoamine oxidase inhibitors (MAOIs) nor, where distress is acute, electroconvulsive therapy (ECT) should be withheld: Unilateral ECT to the nondominant hemisphere minimizes postictal confusion in the already confused (Hall, 1974), though it is probably not so effective as classical full-thickness ECT.

Mania in old age is commonly not expansive but hostile and mixed with depressive elements: It, too, is accordingly often missed, on the basis that the old person is senile and is being obnoxious. It is controllable by phenothiazines and other psychotropic agents, administered with the caution which applies to all drugs in age, and preventable by lithium (Foster et al., 1977) with strict laboratory control, since in the old, blood ion levels can fluctuate widely and suddenly. The diazepam group of drugs should be avoided because of the ease with which they induce confusion. Paraldehyde, nasty as it is, has uses in acute mania dependent on the lack of temptation to continue it prophylactically. Although mania may be mistaken for senility plus ill temper, alcoholic and drug withdrawal can be mistaken for mania; they commonly surface on admission to hospital. Old people are not only more sensitive to drugs, they more easily become dependent on them.

The so-called first-rank symptoms of schizophrenia may all be present in atypical affective disorder, particularly mania. This highly important differential diagnosis is discussed in Chapter 3.

Paranoia in age may accompany mania or depression, or it may stand alone. It needs to be distinguished from well-founded anger, frustration, and suspicion of relatives. At any age, paranoiac ideas serve to fill gaps in the patient's ability to explain experience; they make sense of the senseless. In old age, such ideas often tend to be domestic rather than extravagant, and the blanks they fill are caused by sensory or cortical deficit: People are stealing the mail (since the patient writes no letters, or his friends are dead, he gets none); people are putting dirt in the washing machine (in which the patient forgot to put soap).

The first therapeutic step is to correct sensory deficits and to detect neurological signs, if any. Deafness notoriously predisposes. Paranoiac ideas may be part of a valiant mechanism of denial directed against apraxia, aprosopognosia, or cortical blindness, which the patient may vehemently deny (Anton's syndrome). Here, as always, one must listen carefully to what the patient says. In dementia, the ability to interpret the facial expression of others may be lost or altered (Kurucz et al., 1979). Bizarre experiences such as temporal lobe aurae, which would be recognized in younger people for what they are, may in the old be attributed to paranoia. Reports of odd behavior should be evaluated skeptically: Relatives and nurses interpret as paranoia in the old behavior which in the young would be tolerated. Hidden physical determinants—sensory loss, tinnitus, olfactory hallucinations—should be sought. The paranoid symptoms and the attendant panic may then be controlled by major tranquilizers, in low doses and, since paranoid patients are paranoid about pills and conceal them under the denture for subsequent disposal, in liquid form. Medication must be frank, not surreptitious, or the paranoia will be reinforced with fears of poisoning or ideas of influence. In view of possible hypotensive effects, the patient must be cautioned to take care in getting out of bed during the night and on waking. The complications of prolonged antipsychotic administration in the old include glaucoma, acute retention, extrapyramidal syndrome, and the aggravation of preexisting, tremorless Parkinsonism, but the relief of paranoia is an indication for their cautious use.

The diagnosis of psychotic causes of paranoia is discussed in a subsequent chapter. The main fact to grasp is that it is a wholly nonspecific symptom, associated with many different physical, pharmacological, and pathological agents. It can occur in mania, depression, early dementia and, in susceptible people, without other evidence of psychotic process. The most important element in dealing with its presentation, apart from careful search for nonpsychiatric causes, is to resist the pressure to declare the sufferer irrevocably and irremediably insane, which is often not the case.

The second most common mental problem of the old, especially encountered in general practice, is probably hypochondriasis, at least so far as physician time is concern. Underlying depression must first be excluded, if necessary by a therapeutic trial. After that, students are enjoined to observe three negatives and four positives.

The three negatives are: Don't try to explain to patients the nature of psychosomatic illness—they will go elsewhere. Don't conduct exploratory, and still less punitive, surgery, proctoscopy, and the like. Don't refer the patient.

The four positives are: Investigate adequately but not obsessionally. Agree that the patient is sick and requires treatment. Then give a placebo—for this purpose, an active material such as a tranquilizer should not be used. The traditional "bottle of medicine" possessing trifling activity served as a transitional object and a certificate of permission to be sick, bearing the doctor's name, exhibitable to relatives, and serving as his surrogate to occupy the "interval of therapeutic inactivity." Schedule a definite further appointment. From that point, the therapeutic ingredient is time, devoted to establishing confidence and uncovering personal and situational frustrations against which the symptoms are an appeal for help. In psychotherapy with the old, the tyro and even the experienced therapist, who are accustomed to accepting the transference role of parent, may be disconcerted by reversal or rapid alternation in which they find themselves the target of emotions directed not to parents but to children. They may need to remodel their technique and reexamine their countertransferences, often without warning.

Although hypochondriasis is a common neurotic manifestation in the old, it is also an important sign: The patient's complaints of ill health have been shown (Kay et al., 1966) to be a better index of the four-year mortality rate than initial physician assessment. Complaints of ill health which cannot be substantiated objectively may be a precursor of serious unrelated disease of which neither physician nor patient was aware, besides being the first symptom of major depressive illness in 29% of older depressed patients (D'Alarcon, 1964).

Acute anxiety or panic may occur in the old as in the young. When it does, however, it is more often accompanied by confusion, depression, and added fear on the part of patients that they may be "going out of their mind." The precipitating cause and the predisposition to such reactions may both be obvious, but the attack can be misinterpreted as "senility" or psychosis by those inclined to make such diagnoses readily in old people. Klein (1964) has shown that some anxiety attacks are sympathetic "storms" which have no obvious personality or situational correlates. In young people, some of these are accompaniments of cardiac abnormalities, especially mitral valve prolapse; in the old, acute anxiety and palpitations without obvious stressor causes should be viewed with suspicion and their physical causes considered.

Acute and chronic anxiety reactions and panic states in the old can occur in response to any crisis, but they are specifically associated with a move to unfamiliar surroundings (Hall, 1966), whether this be to the hospital, to a new location, or, in particular, to an apartment that is a mirror image of one they have left. Most of us have experienced confusion on waking in an unfamiliar hotel room. In old age, this is compounded by fear of senility and by sedation, as the loss of time orientation that is normal for persons in the hospital and separated from clocks and calendars can be read as "dementia" in the old. Such panic states respond to normal crisis intervention, sharing, suggestion of coping strategies, and reassurance coupled with help in relearning the environment. So-called minor tranquilizers may be given for one to seven days only, in minimal doses. When tremor, palpitations, and other somatic symtoms are marked and there are no contraindications, propranolol may be preferable (Heiser and De Francisco, 1976) in the control of panic states, but it may of itself cause a severe confusional state in some patients (Kurland, 1979).

Sleep patterns in the old differ from those in the young (see Chapter 7). The typical pattern of normal, intermittent sleep that commonly occurs at home and under quiet, unanxious conditions in old age has figured widely in hypnotic advertisements under the label "geriatric insomnia." It should not be medicated, and staff who awaken older persons from daytime naps should be controlled. The physician should be aware that with the possible exception of chloral hydrate in pediatric doses over short periods, there are no hypnotics which fail to induce some degree of hangover in older subjects, and apparent dementia occasionally responds dramatically to withdrawal of a cherished sleeping pill. Barbiturates in particular can readily induce microsomal enzyme changes, with consequent derangement of calcium metabolism and "senile rickets" presenting as loss of mobility and weakness. They have little or no place in geriatric medicine. Patients and relatives need to be cautioned against over-the-counter medications based on hyoscine and an antihistamine, the effects of which in the old can occasionally be spectacularly deleterious and diagnostically perplexing if not recognized.

Alcohol, as our chief and most threatening drug of abuse, presents problems in old patients, as it does at all ages. Old people "become alcoholic" because of the long latency of confrontation with an alcohol problem, because their tolerance to alcohol declines, and because they abuse alcohol for the first time in age to soften intolerable circumstances and loss of social roles. Others are given drams by relatives to keep them quiet. Alcohol has been lauded in geropsychiatry as a "miracle drug" for palliating the distress of age (Stotsky, 1975). Although the reasons behind this view are clearly argued, to those obliged to deal with its effects, this kind of assertion belongs to the realm of massive social denial which generally surrounds the subject. It would perhaps be true if alcohol, like cocaine, were a controlled substance. For those brought up in the context of this denial, and of the mythology of "social" drinking, permission to continue in a style they have known may be valuable (Chien et al., 1973). On the other hand, alcoholism in old age requires active treatment as at any other age, and old people must be warned of the increased susceptibility to falls and to hangover effects, which even lifelong moderation cannot avoid. More than ever, the older person needs to have his head together.

DEMENTIA

When an old person becomes demented, the cause may be one of the progressive and irreversible processes classed as "senile dementia," but it may equally be covert systemic illness, medication, depression, or endocrine and electrolyte imbalance, since loss of mental acuity and memory in the old is a close equivalent of convulsions in babies or delirium in adults, with the difference that it is far more easily induced. Cataract surgery, for example, is a notorious special precipitant (Summers and Reich, 1979).

Accordingly, when "dementia" is reported, distinction from a secondary, symptomatic, remediable confusional state is the first and most important diagnostic procedure. This applies both to a gradual psychophysical impairment, usually described as "senility" and often taken as natural, and to more dramatic changes confined to intellectual function.

Senile dementia is the layman's image of "old age," and the fear of this destiny does much to pattern gerontophobia in society. It is significant if not epidemic, affecting perhaps a global 10% of persons over 65. The term covers a number of organic diseases characterized by slowly progressive loss of mental capacity, including memory, orientation, and the ability to perform serial tasks. The two leading forms in this continuum are so-called atherosclerotic dementia, which reflects not so much decreased blood flow to the brain as the effect of multiple successive small infarcts, and the Alzheimer group, in which cell loss is prominent. Neither is due to age alone. The infarctive syndrome may possibly be reduced in future age groups by judicious antihypertensive therapy in middle life (and can be precipitated, or aggravated, by injudicious antihypertensive therapy in old age). The Alzheimer group is probably infective, neurochemical, or autoimmune in origin. Compared with the downward sawtooth course of infarctive dementias, that of the Alzheimer group is more smoothly progressive. Drugs have been developed which appear to palliate the course of these conditions (Sathanathan and Gershon, 1975; Lehman and Ban, 1975) but their action is unreliable: The infarctive form sometimes responds to anticoagulant therapy with partial reversal or arrest. These forms of dementia are discussed in detail in Chapter 2. In either case, social and environmental enrichment can enable the patient to live better with the capacity he has. The differential diagnosis is from depressive pseudodementia and symptomatic confusion, from such specific cerebral disorders as normotensive hydrocephalus, and from the effects of medication. The most important pseudodementia seen among the American old is "nursing home disease," a combination of social deprivation, lack of demand, boredom, and chemical restraint by overdoses of tranquilizers given for the convenience of untrained staff and to prevent complaint. This syndrome, which resembles that seen in psychiatrically committed political dissidents living in less-fortunate orders, is remediable by withdrawal of medication and restitution of social responsibilities. Untreated, it passes rapidly into the irremediable dementia which it simulates.

Active treatment of apparent dementia is always justified, whether by therapeutic trial of antidepressants, milieu therapy, or trial of drugs, in view of the course of the untreated disease. Removal of depressive overlay and the mobilization of social interest and intellectual reserves laid fallow by boredom can sometimes effect surprising revivals. At worst, the patient can be helped to live within his cerebral means and given a warm and supportive environment. The need for human contact persists so long as touch can be appreciated and after the loss of memory for faces.

When an old person presents with reported "senility," true dementias are only one of a great range of impairments, many of them treatable, that must be considered. The differential diagnosis of "senility" occupies much of the geriatrician's time and is itself an important test of physician attitude and skill.

2
DIAGNOSIS
AND INVESTIGATION
OF "SENILITY"

"Senility" is the gradual loss of mental or physical function and well-being when this occurs in an elderly person. The distinction between senility and general ill-health depends upon the erroneous belief that age in itself is a sufficient explanation of such changes. In fact, "senility" is to the geriatrician what "failure to thrive" is to the pediatrician—evidence of something wrong which calls for active investigation. In view of the prevalence of genetic diseases revealing themselves in babies, and the rarity of their first appearance in old age, unexplained ill-health is far more commonly idiopathic in pediatric than in geriatric practice. The attitudes of prescientific medicine to the major infectious diseases of infancy in some respects resembles the attitude by which senility is considered as a diagnosis, in that prescientific medicine attributed to age (in that case infancy) those phenomena which in adults would be recognized as specific pathologies. In the case of the old, these are specific pathologies in which the signs and symptoms of textbook medicine, which is predominantly the medicine of adult and middle life, are muted or altered by aging and obscured by the persisting misconception that disability can be attributed to chronology alone.

Old people do not in fact become weak, frail, immobile, or demented through any common or universal change coupled to chronologic age in the way that loss of hair pigment is coupled. Their liability to pathologies, in particular multiple pathologies, increases, and although 75% of persons over 65 describe themselves as "well," about 86% suffer from one or more chronic conditions, which may be minor in their impact on function; the 10–15% who are seriously "unwell" commonly have more than one such condition. In these evidently ill patients, "senility" is no more than a slightly derogatory term for the physical and mental concomitants of chronic and explainable ill-health. When it presents alone, and in the absence of any such history, it means an ongoing loss of function from an occult cause, which in a younger person would lead to intensive investigation, but which in the old, is treated as something to be expected. The main achievement of geriatric medicine, and the main requirement for its effective practice on the European model, is the liquidation of this erroneous belief.

HOW "SENILITY" PRESENTS

"Senility" is not a complaint of the patient but a report by relatives or custodians of an old person. The patient may complain of weakness, loss of activity, or confusion and attribute these changes to age. In either event, the factual basis is that there is a change in the patient, so that he can no longer do what he recently did. In popular use, "senility" refers to loss of intellectual function or even to resentful or inconvenient behavior, which, however justified by the setting, can be charitably attributed to such loss.

How does "senility" present in our office? The following case is a good example:

The father of a distinguished geriatrician was an active and feisty old man in his mid eighties, twice a widower, and a wayward pursuer of his own concerns. His son was notified by an alarmed family that "Dad was failing." He sat in a chair, from which he now had difficulty in rising; he no longer showed interest in women or in food. More seriously, he had three times parked his car, forgotten where he had parked it, and reported it stolen. On the first two occasions, the police were tolerant; on the third, they suggested that the patient might have outlived his eligibility for a driving licence. A local practitioner diagnosed "old age." On examination, the old man was rational but a little confused, and the fire had gone out of him. He was also losing weight and experiencing fatigue on moving about.

I will return to this case in a moment, because the outcome is instructive. The patient was fortunate in having a geriatrician in the family. In less affluent or less supportive circumstances, he would have risked admission to a custodial institution, sedation in response to his anger at the procedure, and early death from medical neglect or the civilized equivalent of black magic—not uncommon outcomes of symptomatic disorientation in the old when "senility" is treated as a diagnosis.

Although this popular reading of senility covers the actual symptoms—confusion and memory loss, hostile or difficult behavior, and dementia—which point to wholly different probable causes, equally common modes of presentation are weakness and loss of mobility in the absence of obvious cause such as arthritic pain, often described as "getting frail" or "going off his feet," fatigue, and a general lack of appetency, including anorexia, loss of interest in events, and "giving up" on life—again often charitably interpreted by relatives as a fitting and even natural preparation for the cue to leave the stage. Often the onset of this downward slope in the life of the patient is presaged by a series of unexplained falls ("premonitory falls" in geriatric parlance). These may represent not only neurological disorders such as unrecognized Parkinsonism, or ingravescent stroke, but also one of the common presentations in old age of heart attack, heart failure, chest or urinary infection, or the equally ingravescent side effects of medication.

The common thread in all these "senile" manifestations is that in old age, the presentation of major illness is commonly nonspecific. Moreover, the popular reading of senility as "second childishness" cannot be separated from the physical pathologies that occur in age, because confusion, memory loss, and behavioral and mood changes are often increasingly symptomatic in older patients, as delirium is symptomatic of febrile illness in the young—the difference being that in old age, they may be the only symptoms.

"SENILITY" AS A MENTAL SYMPTOM

The most common disorders of intellect in old age are not dementias, but symptomatic clouding of consciousness and endogenous depression with approximately equal frequency. Endogenous depression in the old may present as hypochondria or pseudodementia, may be accompanied by loss of activity and interest, and can itself impair physical health. It is also treatable by appropriate antidepressant therapy. Symptomatic confusion, memory loss, or agitation can result from any silent infection, cerebrovascular or coronary occlusion, electrolyte disturbance from any cause, and the effects of medication. In contrast to the major organic dementias, these symptomatic changes are often (though not always) less gradual in onset, and they are transient if the cause is removed before grave physical and social damage has been done: No true dementia comes on in a matter of days or weeks. The major disease process may differ from its typical adult form in being painless (coronary occlusion), afebrile (pneumonia, pyelitis), and attended by minimal signs.

Symptomatic mental illness in the old, whether it presents as memory loss, acute confusion, or apathy, is usually recognized for what it is when it occurs in the presence of obvious sickness, but unfortunately, this is often not the case. Mental symptoms of what is in fact minor delirium presenting as the only evidence of disorder can be the first or sole evidence of pneumonia, urinary infection, uremia, congestive heart failure, minor cerebral infarction without other gross neurological signs, diabetic ketosis or hypoglycemia, and hypothermia, to which old persons living in cold areas and inadequate housing are especially prone. This last condition appears to be more common, or more often recognized, in Europe. In all these cases, the myth of "senility" may lead the incautious to miss the underlying pathology—a serious matter, because where this is treatable, mental function usually recovers completely. So long as the mental association between "age" and "dementia" persists, the minimal increase in respiratory rate of afebrile pneumonia or the presence of urinary infection can be missed. The diagnosis of Valium deficiency and other injudicious interventions directed to quiet the "demented" patient can add to the mischief. Institutionalization in a custodial "home" is in itself a potent cause of nocturnal confusion, especially in those already sick, and treatment by chemical restraint constitutes an unintentional form of euthanasia in a patient whose mental confusion was curable by a doctor with minimal geriatric training.

Next to infection, the commonest cause of senility presenting with confusion is medication. For this reason, the first step taken in its investigation by European geriatricians is the "plastic bag test," cited in Chapter 1—the assembling in one bag of all the substances, prescribed, bought, and borrowed, which the patient is ingesting. These may number several dozen, and rarely number less than five or six. The second is the cessation of all medication which is not life-sustaining. Let me go back to the case cited above:

> The geriatrician's father received a careful physical examination, which revealed no sign of infection or any other of the common physical causes of his condition. He denied taking any medication. Diligent enquiry, however, revealed that after the death of his first wife, many years before, he had been unable to sleep, and since that time, he had taken a single butobarbital tablet every night. When his second wife died, five years ago, he again could not sleep, and added a single nightly Quaalude tablet. This trifling amount of medication was stopped, despite his protests. Within ten days, his activity and appetency returned, he ate well, he pursued comely women, and he never again "mislaid" his car. His strength and posture also greatly improved with the removal of mild osteomalacia caused by the microsomal-inductive effect of the barbiturate, from which he had been suffering.

SENILE WEAKNESS

Physical strength, in athletic terms, normally declines with age, but such a decline is also normally gradual. The patient adjusts to it, and weakness of rapid onset, similar to that experienced in earlier life after a severe illness, is always symptomatic. Weakness may cover increasing dyspnea, or clinically predictable conditions such as anemia, but in the old, rather less familiar causes may operate. The weakness of spontaneous or drug-induced osteomalacia (senile rickets) is one such cause; another is the myopathy of silent hyperthyroidism. Excessive secretion of T3, T4, or both can occur in the aged, with or without exophthalmos, restlessness, and thyroid enlargement; in the "apathetic" form of thyrotoxicosis, weakness may be severe enough to inhibit even leisurely movement. Bahemuka and Hodkinson (1975) found an incidence of 2.25% unrecognized hypothyroidism and over 1% unrecognized hyperthyroidism in aged subjects, both presenting with the nonspecific syndrome of "failure to thrive."

Both weakness and confusion can result from heart failure, either following a painless coronary episode or as the convergence on an aging myocardium of several trivial stresses which can combine to induce decompensation (Pomerance, 1972). Weakness alone characterizes the sodium depletion of inappropriate antidiuretic hormone secretion (SIADH), which can complicate, or be the presenting symptom of, infection, malignancy, and myxoedema (Bartter and Schwartz, 1967). Sodium depletion is also readily induced by the officious use of diuretics, one of the most common medications in the old.

Weakness can also mask the stiffness of Parkinsonism, which can occur without evident tremor but responds to L-dopa. Hodkinson (1976) emphasizes the importance of Wartenberg's head-drop sign (Wartenburg, 1952) as a test for rigidity. The treatment of hypertension in old age, if based on criteria appropriate for a younger patient, can induce a form of "senility" (Jackson et al, 1976), compounded of weakness due to hypokalemia or hyponatremia, loss of confidence from postural hypotension, lowering of mood by ganglion blocking agents, and interference with sexual function from the same cause. These side effects of many antihypertensive therapies can render the cure more onerous than the disease even at earlier ages, but their effects are particularly prominent in the old, in whom treatment of nominal hypertension can severely disorder both well-being and brain function.

SENILE MEMORY LOSS

In common with other responses, recall becomes slower with age. This effect, which troubled Thomas Jefferson and led him to argue against a life term for the Presidency, is most prominent in those least mentally active but causes most anxiety to the intellectual. It is, however, benign and nonprogressive. Severe deterioration of memory can herald the major dementias, but equally common or commoner causes are undiagnosed myxoedema and hangover due to the use, even in normally acceptable doses, of any sedative drug. Alcohol, even in moderate amount, can lead to an amnestic syndrome. There are no "minor tranquilizers" in geriatrics, nor should the normal later-life pattern of sleep be medicated; it must, however, be distinguished from the early waking characteristic of depressive illness.

ABNORMAL BEHAVIOR

Behavior which is odd or objectionable in the young is interpreted as "senility" in the old, by common consent of the culture. The young man who assaults little girls is seen as psychopathic; the old man who does so, even when his access to more normal sexual gratification is restricted by lack of opportunity or by infirmity, is described as "senile."

Persons whose behavior was odd in youth may become odder with age as the pressure of societal rejection comes to bear on them. Paranoia at any age is cover for unexplainable experiences—in the old, these may include the attempt to cover sensory losses such as deafness, cortical blindness, or symptomatic amnesias. It may also express the psychic recognition of the hostility of relatives. Anomic behavior and self-neglect can represent gradual increase in confusion and weakness from remediable or irremediable causes. Sometimes this loss of ability to tend to oneself is compounded by personal pride, which makes the patient unwilling to let others see him or her in a neglected condition. The idea that old people are more commonly lonely than young, except after bereavement, may well be exaggerated as a cause of depression. Where isolation and depression coexist in the old, the isolation and neglect are more commonly results of endogenous depression than causes of reactive depression.

Loss of morale is inherent in the concept of senility. At all other ages and in all other conditions, society, while it may not be supportive of disability, tends to support by its attitude the attempt of the patient to cope. In age, the pressure is in the other direction—to accept the fitness, propriety, and naturalness of decline, and to bury the older person, healthy or ailing, prematurely by a process of social devaluation. Hardy individuals in reasonable health can resist this pressure, but any symptoms of impairment from whatever cause tend to excite in the elderly invalid, however robust his self-image, the anxiety that society may be right after all. It is in age that we most often see the syndrome of self-willed death (Hodkinson, 1976; Milton, 1973) otherwise confined to those who believe in the efficacy of sorcery. One function of the geriatrician is accordingly as a breaker of spells cast by the folklore of old age.

THE INVESTIGATION OF "SENILITY"

The investigation of "senility" resolves itself into the careful search for the underlying pathology, the removal of iatrogenic disease where present, and the healing, in patient, relatives, and the physician, of the sorcery wrought by the assumption of causeless infirmity as a feature of old age.

The minimal exclusionary approach to senility includes proper history, a full physical examination carried out with patience—no simple matter where confusion or deafness limit cooperation—with special attention to infections and to the signs, often minimal, of endocrine and metabolic disorder, and a battery of tests directed to the known causes of nonspecific illness. For such a battery, Hodkinson suggests (Hodkinson, 1976) chest x-ray, with attention to signs of infection, pulmonary edema, neoplasm, and bony changes, including fractures and Looser's zones in the scapula; Coulter S blood count; BUN and electrolytes, serum albumin and globulin, calcium, phosphates and alkaline phosphatase, a random blood sugar, T4 and T3 uptake, and routine urinalysis. To these should be added thorough enquiry into, and reevaluation of, all medications without exception. This should be carried out with reference to a geriatric textbook, not the manufacturer's literature, since the list of precautions and side effects required by the FDA contains no special reference to drug hazards in age. All medication not evidently life sustaining may well be withdrawn, with due attention to possible effects of sudden discontinuance and interaction between retained and withdrawn drugs, e.g., through loss of ribosomal induction. When investigation is complete and symptoms have remitted or been explained, only those medications clearly indicated should be reinstated, and those should not exceed four or five in number, however numerous the pathologies identified. Sedatives, antihypertensives, and diuretics are the most abused drugs in older persons. They are rarely or never indicated for prolonged use.

Headache in the old, a frequent psychiatric referral, may be due to most of the causes that operate in the young, but two commonly misdiagnosed and specifically geriatric causes are Paget's disease and temporal arteritis. Arteritis is a medical emergency calling for energetic treatment with steroids, because of the high risk of blindness. It should be suspected in any elderly person with persistent unilateral headache. It can be confused with herpes zoster and with migraine. Palpable temporal arteries and signs of polymyalgia should be sought, the fundi inspected, and arterial biopsy performed. This is a condition in which minimal physical signs accompanying headache can be missed, especially in the polysymptomatic patient, and the problem dismissed as "functional" until sight in one eye deteriorates. When this occurs, steroid medication will not as a rule reverse the retinal damage, although it may prevent the loss of the other eye, which often follows in the untreated case. The pain of Paget's disease is cranial, and the patient may complain that his or her hats are now too small. Migraine, contrary to popular belief, can persist in the old, both in its typical and atypical forms, including a form confined to aurae and associated with depersonalization and atypical depression. In any migraine syndrome, the character of the attacks can change. Unusual aurae may give rise to anxiety and must be distinguished from premonitory TIAs: Motor weakness, except in hemiplegic migraine, is virtually never migrainous, but sensory aurae may be. Waking at night with rapidly transient dysphasia or a scotoma after a period of REM sleep is generally migrainous, especially if it leaves residual unilateral headache, but any first attack of ischemic-like symptoms in the old should be viewed with suspicion. Migraine may begin de novo in the old, but much more often it will have been present throughout life.

Psychotherapy, in the form of an opportunity to discuss the experience and hardships of aging, if not with the physician, then with any sympathetic and undemeaning listener, forms part of the treatment of every geriatric patient in our society, whether their problems are "psychiatric" or not. A physician who cannot spare the time for at least one extended interview of this sort with every senior patient should probably be practicing pathology rather than clinical medicine, but the further support of the patient can then be transferred to others, including nurses, students, and social workers, to whom the patient should be courteously introduced by the physician in charge, so that the transference can be transferred (rather than the sensitive patient "shunted off"). Support both of the patient and of the patient's relatives by a discussion-type therapy group, led by a skilled individual, is an invaluable help when it can be organized. For the justifiably bored and angry, introduction to a militant seniors' advocacy organization can sometimes work a remarkable transformation.

In the presence of mental changes, it is clearly necessary to distinguish between symptomatic confusion, psychosis, and true dementia. The gradual onset of degenerative brain syndrome and the stepwide ingravescence of "atherosclerotic" (infarctive) dementia are characteristic where they occur, but symptomatic confusion can also be chronic or episodic. Goldfarb (1971) stresses the use of his mental status questionnaire (Kahn, Pollack, and Goldfarb, 1961) in conjunction with Bender's double simultaneous stimulation (face—hand) test in detecting pseudodementia, but psychometric tests cannot always discriminate reversible from irreversible mischief, and the proper approach is exclusionary, since even in the presence of some organic impairment, intercurrent illness can produce reversible exacerbation and make the difference between impaired performance and frank dementia.

ROLE OF THE FAMILY

The mythology of the extended family as the natural and ideal support mechanism for the old may cause the physician to miss the frequent but unwelcome fact that "senility" can be precipitated by family collusion as certainly as by a bad nursing home. The family can indeed be a support mechanism for the patient, but it is also a mutual-support mechanism for the neuroses and character disorders of its members, and the theater in which they are acted out. In such a situation, the old person, often the bottom man on the totem pole, may have to be rescued from overprotection, smiling persecution, childrenization, gradual euthanasia, or even physical abuse. All the adult pathologies that are inflicted on children, from violence to the double bind, are quite often inflicted on the old. The victim may react by fear, querulousness, tantrums, or alcoholism, or by suicide, but where physical illness is present, he or she may also react by regression, by becoming helpless and incontinent, and by using guilt over obligation as a weapon.

Family pathology is far easier to recognize in the less-common cases, where an old person shows neglect, is starved, or has bruises, than in the "smiling" variety, where the invalid may be treated with assiduous care and veiled hostility. It is possible with practice to develop a sixth sense that all is not well, especially when the next of kin shows no willingness to admit that the care of the patient is burdensome (for this reason if for no other, house calls, if not by the geriatrician, then by a skilled social worker or public health nurse, are mandatory when a supposedly "senile" old person lives with relatives).

A not uncommon manifestation in geriatric practice is the "Jekyll and Hyde" syndrome (Boyd and Woodman, 1978). An old person living with a devoted but often unwilling relative is a helpless and incontinent invalid at home. On hospital admission, the patient rapidly improves, becomes continent, rational, and mobile, and within days of discharge, relapses into complete dependence again, the aggrieved relative remarking that the discharge was incomprehensible because the patient is no better. This cycle can be repeated many times. It represents a competition in family psychopathology—aggressive dependence vs. denied hostility—and is best terminated by intermittent care (one week on, one week off). The Jekyll and Hyde syndrome characteristically occurs when only the dependent patient and the entrapped caretaker are involved: Introduction of other people into the contest may moderate its violence, to the relief of both contestants.

The best quick index of the likelihood of such an overlay, bearing in mind that caring for an old relative is invariably and realistically stressful, is whether the patient is treated as an ailing adult or as a child. Where sickness is severe, some practical role reversal between parent and child is normal and inevitable, but the adulthood of the patient is respected. Much can be learned by noting how the old person is spoken to and handled.

TESTING THE MENTAL CAPACITY OF THE OLD (See Chapter 5)

An old person subjected to mental testing is defensive. Aware of the social expectation of senility, less accustomed to what appear to be pointless exercises than the IQ-ridden generations which grew up after them, and easily time stressed, the old may approach mental tests in much the same frame of mind as a solitary black pupil in a school full of hostile whites whose teacher has prefaced the exercise with a racist discourse on the mental superiority of Anglo-Saxons. That they require to be reassured is an understatement: The magnitude of the increment in scores after administration of a beta-blocking agent (Eisdorfer et al., 1970) is concrete evidence of this need.

Slowing which affects the majority of physical responses is a normal consequence of age. Normal old people do not operate quickly, and they react badly to time stress, taking refuge in confusion or negativism. It is a privilege of age to close the door. Many a hearing aid has been ordered because, on the day of the audiometrist's visit, the patient was not talking to anyone. In modern society with its high informational flux, old people may be chronically hustled to the point of confusion, and the timing scale of any task used in testing must be modified to exclude this spurious cause of underperformance.

Since confusion is so often symptomatic, it must be looked for in every geriatric examination. On the other hand, a healthy older person, confronted on admission by a doctor young enough to be his son who asks him if he knows what year it is, can be pardoned for terminating cooperation at that point. Orientation can be determined in a wholly unthreatening manner, however, since many items of the standard Hodkinson (1972) short inventory come within the scope of normal case taking—name, age, birthplace, address, name of next of kin, occupation or former occupation, and even the time of the appointment, the name of the physician, and the time of day. The patient can be asked to remember an address or phrase for five-minute recall; other essential tests, such as counting backward, are best incorporated into the physical CNS examination. Only if disorientation appears on this inventory need its extent be pursued; both mental state and the presence and nature of aphasia or memory defect can be established from conversation. When they have been cited by relatives, they can be referred to the patient in specific questions. Occasional episodes of confusion are terrifying and their occurrence is likely to be volunteered, whereas even the apparently caring narration of relatives should be viewed with insightful skepticism.

ATTITUDES TO THE OLD PATIENT

The physician's examination of the old, like his response to an avowedly homosexual patient, merits close self-examination. If it is based on unrecognized anxiety or on hostile or patronizing attitudes, these will be projected, however bland the approach, for the nerves of the old are as raw to perceive prejudice as those of a persecuted minority to sense bigotry. It is helpful, perhaps, to recall the following: an old person both is and feels himself or herself to be the same person as in youth. Others are seen to change, but not we ourselves, and it is the response of others which changes, from valuation to devaluation, from conventional social respect to impatience. Conversation proceeds as if the old person were not there. Waiters will ask not the patient but the son or daughter, "Does he take cream in his coffee?" So while we remain inwardly as we were, our social surroundings and our juniors increasingly treat us as objects. The physician who not only knows this but empathizes, and projects his empathy, will practice geriatric psychiatry with success. It is, after all, reasonable to work on those nosogenic attitudes in society, if only to protect ourselves grown old.

3

MAJOR PSYCHOSES

With the exception of "involutional depression," psychosis does not often begin de novo in persons over 65. When it does, the physician is probably wiser not to be overconcerned with the niceties of psychiatric nomenclature, as between "late paraphrenia," paranoid schizophrenia, and other categories, since these exist for convenience only and have little bearing on treatment or prognosis. The physician's most important tasks are to exclude physical causes and to consider the possibility of affective disorder. The treatment of thought disorder and of paranoia is symptomatic, with antipsychotic drugs, but the possibility of underlying depression or mania makes radical treatment, and prevention of recurrence, possible. Because there is only a limited number of ways in which mental disorder can express itself, confusion, thought disorder, ideas of influence, and paranoic manifestations are best regarded as nonspecific symptoms or final common paths. The most critical pointers when gross physiological disturbances have been excluded are family history (schizophrenic and affective family histories do not interchange, although both types of illness may have been present in a pedigree; these two forms of mental pathology accordingly "breed true") and previous personality, which may have to be indirectly assessed, e.g., from marital or work record. Previous physical illness should be reviewed, because it may indicate cyclicity and cover a history of recurrent depression or excitement: In bipolar illness, mania may have appeared only as exaggerated well-being unless judgment was much impaired.

In spite of intensive propaganda to the contrary, it is still rational to regard major psychoses as changes in self-experience mediated by changes in cerebral chemistry. The wholly existential view (that they are learned behaviors arising from adverse parent-child interaction) was rejected by Freud, and is supported only by evidence which could equally indicate the high vulnerability of some individuals and, very probably, their failure in early childhood to return the "passwords" necessary to further normal parent—child bonding. The experience of major depression differs qualitatively from grief, and that of schizophrenia from the customary posture of other persons in the culture. In spite of this, overt illness is precipitated in predisposed people by life experience. Surprisingly enough, this kind of precipitation is no more common in the old than in the young, although ego-threatening stresses multiply with age. Post (1968) found that depressive illness in persons over 60 was preceded by a few days by major stress (death of a spouse, illness, disorientation following a move) in about 75% of cases, but as Post himself points out (Post, 1978), studies of depressives aged 18—65 (Brown et al., 1975) also show a 75—86% incidence of similar precipitation in depressive illness. More significantly, precipitating factors could be identified in 41% of severely psychotic depressives as opposed to only 29% of those whose condition was diagnosed as "neurotic" (i.e., nonpsychotic) depression (Post, 1978). However gross the cultural attack on the old, the general increased incidence of depressive illness with age is probably due equally to increased vulnerability of affective mechanisms produced by the changes which occur in significant neuroamines: The role of cultural deprivation and personal loss is that, given the chemical vulnerability, the precipitants are there.

AFFECTIVE DISORDER

The fact that both cyclical and intermittent severe depressions can occur at any age, with or without obvious provoking circumstances, may obscure the fact that "severe depressions are essentially disorders of later life" (Post, 1978). The traditional view has sometimes been of "endogenous" (i.e., apparently unprovoked) depressions, sometimes cyclical, sometimes alternating with mania, sometimes "atypical" (associated with other mental symptoms such as obsessions or paranoid phenomena), and "neurotic" depressions in which anxiety was more evident than retardation and the more severe manifestations (nihilistic ideas, delusions, suicide) less prominent. Although sharply cyclical cases do appear to have their own natural history, affective illness appears to be a final common path. Its components (the relative prevalence of depression, anxiety, apathy, or somatic complaints), its polarity (depression vs. mania), and the infusion of "schizophrenic" features such as ideas of influence and hallucinations form a continuum.

If depression is scored on the Zung self-assessment questionnaire, many older people score as mildly depressed in the absence of any specific pathology because of the bias imposed by the questionnaire's emphasis on usefulness, activity, and the like—all attributes which are socially limited in the old.

The incidence of true depressive episodes in older persons has never been accurately estimated, but it is high. Moreover, first depressive episodes requiring hospital admission are at their maximum between ages 50 and 65, and first attacks become rare only after age 80 (Post, 1968). Besides these evident attacks in which distress is obviously mental and suicide is an overt threat, lesser but no less potentially dangerous depressions are the most common and most underdiagnosed psychiatric emergency in geriatric practice.

The task of the geriatrician is not, in most cases, to attempt by clinical means to differentiate endogenous from reactive or neurotic depression, but to be vigilant for any depressive symptoms, whether intelligible in the patient's situation or not, to suspect depression in somatic complaints not otherwise explained, and to treat affective symptoms as a potential emergency. Grief and distress are not pathological when appropriate, but in view of the fact that even grossly psychotic depression is commonly triggered, their duration and their content must be watched; important signs are ideas of worthlessness, especially when accompanied by early waking and loss of interest, and excessive duration.

A patient who shows unexplained dysphoria and grief or unhappiness of long duration is depressed rather than sad if four or more of the following indices are present:

anorexia

weight loss

insomnia

psychomotor retardation

loss of self-esteem

inappropriate guilt

impaired concentration and memory

undue fatigue

recurrent or occasional thoughts of death and suicide

feelings of the worthlessness of life

loss of usual interests, including libido

The difficulty of diagnosis is compounded by the fact that some or all of these may appear to be natural or explicable in an older person, so that the pathological resetting of affect becomes evident to patient and doctor only when treatment or spontaneous recovery terminates the depressive episode. Moreover, in our culture, denial of unhappiness is a social pose ("fortitude," being uncomplaining), so that somatic complaints, which are culturally permitted, may be substituted. The stereotype of aging as a period of illness may also make an older person consider unaccustomed dysphoria to be normal.

Recurrent late-life depressions are almost invariably complicated by other concomitants of age such as physical illness, losses, and the recrudescence of life-long anxieties, but they remain treatable and may respond well, in spite of realistic sources of fear and sadness.

Mr. K. was a 90-year-old bachelor and a World War I veteran who was born in Scotland and had a strict Nonconformist background. He was admitted in severe depression, deeply concerned about failing eyesight from cataract, the appearance of a skin cancer, recurrence of peptic ulcer pain, and insomnia.

His first depressive attack occurred at age 51. Without precipitating cause, he had become extremely agitated. In fear of becoming insane, he had thrown himself down a staircase and fractured his spine in two places. He survived the injury, and the depression remitted without specific treatment, but he remained three years in the hospital. After a depression-free interval, during which he was treated for recurrent duodenal ulcer, he was readmitted four years later, preoccupied with feelings of unworthiness, anxiety over masturbation, and rumination over his deafness, which he attributed to "self-abuse." The attack was brief and again resolved without medication. At age 88, he was again admitted with milder depression and agitation, which were not of psychotic proportions. Small doses of chlorpromazine and doxepin rapidly reduced his agitation and aborted the attack.

Mr. K. neither smoked nor drank. He enjoyed Saturday night dances until the age of 82. He had not married because eligible women had not come his way, and he twice caught gonorrhea from less eligible and more accessible ones. He was filled with regrets—for not having bettered himself, for not having taken advantage of the California real estate boom, for not having fathered a family—and with fears—of cancer, blindness, and above all loss of his wits through senility. These somatic anxieties were realistic, although at 90 he was alert, oriented, highly intelligent, and, in view of his medical history, remarkably robust. Besides his ulcer, he had had a nephrectomy for renal carcinoma at 69, partial thyroidectomy to remove a "cold" nodule at 76, anginal attacks, with arrhythmia, controlled by nitroglycerin and digoxin, deafness, cataract, a squamous carcinoma of the temple, extensive seborrheic keratosis suggesting Leser-Trélat's sign, and hepatomegaly for which he declined laparotomy. In spite of this multiple pathology and the realistic awareness that death must be faced, his depression rapidly dissipated with doxepin and the prospect of help with his sensory deficits. He derived much comfort from the support of the staff and fellow patients and from "reminiscence therapy." We had the impression that for the first time in his life, he was reviewing himself without fear or guilt. He died a year later, of cardiac arrest.

In contrast to the frequent treatability of depressions of late initial onset, however, recurrent lifelong cyclical depression may also become refractory as the patient approaches old age. Psychiatrists of the past century were familiar with the phenomenon of late, unrelieved depression which showed no sign of spontaneous resolution. Such cases are still with us, and they present in the geropsychiatric clinic, often ending in chronicity or suicide when antidepressants or even ECT, which had apparently terminated earlier attacks, fail to work. Some patients in whom, during old age, tricyclics fail when earlier they worked will be found on blood-level measurement to have toxic drug levels at ordinary doses (Appelbaum et al., 1979) and to recover on lowered doses.

The basic pathophysiology of truly refractory depression is probably neurochemical—a loss of the capacity of the mood-setting mechanism to rebound, either spontaneously or with therapy. Drift in brain catecholamine levels is an established feature of aging (Finch, 1976), as are changes in response to thyroid-stimulating hormone (TSH), but psychological and situational factors—loss of futurity and social role, physical deficits, bereavement, and sometimes residuals from suicidal attempts—also combine to make the depressive affect and the somatic concerns realistic. The therapist faces a dilemma, in that it is impossible to deal with these real losses by ventilation and support while the psychotic state persists, and often impossible to elevate mood by drugs or ECT: Each new failure with a previously successful therapy then tends to aggravate the patient's despair. The relation of situation to chemistry is, of course, not confined to age and explains the fact that most frankly psychotic depressions are triggered by some situational element. It seems rational to work as far as possible with supportive psychotherapy within the limits of mood and without singing songs to a heavy heart. Aging requires fortitude of the robust, and that fortitude is beyond the powers of those whose affect is easily disturbed. In assessing whether therapies are really ineffective, it is important to remember that during an attack, depressed patients often underrate the success of past efforts (they may say that several previous courses of ECT did nothing for them, while the physician notes made at the time suggest otherwise). Moreover, patients in a "given up, giving up" state of mind may fail to take, or refuse, medication, because of side effects, somatic preoccupations (obstructed bowels, inner emptiness, inability to swallow), as a hindrance to their growing counterphobic anxiety to hasten what they see as their inevitable and timely death, or because the drug selected makes them feel worse (see Table 3.1). Obsessional and guilty thoughts over trifles, rumination, and preoccupation with real or imaginary life-threatening illness are common and are linked with a comprehensible hostility to doctors whose magic has run out. Psychotherapy may be stymied by withdrawal and refusal to discuss these preoccupations, and sometimes by complete mutism.

Whatever the biochemical flaw in such cases, late depression of this sort invariably calls up all the patient's previously laid ghosts in a magnified form. The only sensible treatment plan seems to be constant and active review of antidepressant therapies, with special reference to adequacy of dose and plasma levels, and of ECT as an option. If these fail, unconventional (amphetamines, thyroxin, androgens) or frankly heroic (combined MAOI and tricyclic) therapies should at least be considered with an eye to any clinical pointers: There are small subgroups of depression in which they occasionally seem to work (see page 32). It may be necessary also to substitute directive sorcery for simple support: The patient is given an amytal interview to break down mutism, and strong directive suggestion is aimed at guilt, somatic preoccupation, and hopelessness. The patient has little to lose and some hope of amelioration. If social interaction and physical activity can be established, medical treatment sometimes regains its efficacy. Intractable depression represents perhaps the only instance in medicine when it is always better to do something than nothing.

TABLE 3.1. Table of the Tricyclic Antidepressants

Generic names	Registered brand names	Usual daily dosage (mg)	Geriatric starting dose (mg)	Specific characteristics
Amitriptyline	Elavil Endep	75–300	25	Sedating; most anticholinergic; probably the most toxic
Desipramine	Norpramin Pertofrane	75–200	25	The least anticholinergic
Doxepin	Adapin Sinequan	75–300	25	Commonly used in elderly, cardiac, or debilitated patients (validity?), least guanethidine inhibition, sedating
Imipramine	Imavate Janimine Presamine Tofranil SK-Pramine	75–300	25	The standard antidepressant
Nortriptyline	Aventyl Pamelor	75–100	25	Used in lower dosages
Protriptyline	Vivactil	20–60	5–10	The most potent on a per milligram basis; not sedating

Comments:

Contraindications: acute myocardial infarction, allergy, first trimester pregnancy.

Use with caution: organic brain syndromes, epilepsy, pregnancy, children, elderly, cardiovascular disease, schizophrenia, thyroid disease, glaucoma, urinary retention (e.g., benign prostatic hypertrophy), patients receiving electroconvulsive therapy.

Warnings: drug and alcohol interactions; side effects, especially sedation and anticholinergic symptoms.

Most common anticholinergic side effects: dry mouth, blurry vision, constipation.

Other anticholinergic side effects: exaggeration of glaucoma predisposition, mydriasis, urinary stasis, sexual dysfunction, tachycardia, delirium.

Mild anticholinergic side effects can be useful as guideposts to the approach of a therapeutic dose level and used for their placebo effects, showing the patient that the "medicine is beginning to work."

Maintenance dose levels should be at or near one-half to one-third of the peak level.

Very, very lethal in suicide overdoses.

Tricyclics potentiate: anticholinergic drugs (e.g., antiparkinsonians, scopolamine), major and minor tranquilizers, sedatives, alcohol, sympathomimetics.

With monoamine oxidase inhibitors, hypertensive reactions have been reported.

Tricyclics reportedly inactivate the effects of: some anticonvulsants, guanethidine (Ismelin), rauwolfia alkaloids (should never be used in depressed patients).

Tricyclics reportedly are inactivated to some degree by estrogens, smoking, sedatives, alcohol and possibly phenytoin (Dilantin).

Some experts doubt that doxepin is any safer than other tricyclics.

Modified from Lippmann, S. (1978).

Neurotic depression, if severe enough to copy psychosis, would have to mean depression as a way of life pursued for secondary gains—control over others, revenge, self-punishment, and the availability of suicide threats whenever the patient is frustrated. The difficulty of establishing the diagnosis depends on the fact that any patient liable to severe mood swings will incorporate them into the manipulation of life conflicts. Accordingly, however gross the manipulative element, it does not exclude response to tricyclics, because there is usually more than a grain of endogenous depression in the mass of symptomatology. Such patients may get shorter shrift than the frank psychotic because of countertransference reactions to their querulousness and manipulative behavior, and because they depress, and often express hostility to, the therapist. It is necessary to gauge how far the prospect of cure is itself threatening, avoid attacking the secondary gains, and wait until mood improves with drug treatment. If it does improve, group therapy or family therapy may be the least threatening way of reshaping the patient's dependence on his or her symptoms for power and protection. A depression cannot be assumed to be wholly behavioral because it responds to psychotherapy alone: Endogenous depressions tend toward spontaneous recovery, and the therapy in use at the time may be credited, especially if it has been recently changed. There are, however, chronically unhappy people who are not helped by antidepressants but are helped by psychotherapy—the term "depressive neurotic reaction" (abandoned in the latest nomenclature) presumably indicates cases of this kind.

By contrast, the "borderline" patient, or habitual overreacter, whose response to stress is multifarious but always excessive or irrational, has been shown to do extremely well on low-dose neuroleptics (Brinkley et al., 1979), which render self-comprehension and self-critical psychotherapy possible. There will be patients of this kind whose instability has never really been addressed before they reach old age, and who form a geriatric subgroup. Such patients will be an exception to the general maxim of not giving maintenance antipsychotics in old age except to the frankly schizophrenic or demented. Determining if a difficult and chronically upset and upsetting patient is "borderline" rather than neurotic might best be undertaken by way of a brief clinical trial. Where antipsychotics work, they transform the situation, in contrast to minor tranquilizers, which tend only to postpone a diagnosis. How many "neurotics" subjected to lifelong historical psychotherapy owe their vulnerability to a basically unstable neurotransmitter balance only future investigation will show.

MANAGEMENT OF DEPRESSION

Every older patient in whom depression is suspected must be (a) asked specifically whether they have contemplated suicide, (b) asked specifically whether they believe themselves to have cancer or some other terminal illness, and (c) admitted to hospital if there is any doubt concerning the risk of self-injury; evasive answers or negativism should be interpreted as grounds for doubt. Asking the patient frankly about suicide will not precipitate it, and may even prevent it. Hospital admission raises difficult problems. Even by the undepressed old, hospitals may be seen as places from which one never again comes out. Patients with a history of past attacks of depression (who, during recurrence, frequently remember the affect only of the attacks, not of the intervals of normality) may view any psychiatric institution with loathing and despair. For either of these groups, skillful reassurance and support are necessary: Given these, consent can usually be obtained, on the basis that the attack can be stopped, but this is a promise on which the doctor must deliver, or depression may become despair. For this reason, the latency of effect must be explained to the patient if tricyclics are given, and frequent support from nursing staff and the physician must be organized while medication is being given time to act. A time limit should finally be set: "If you are no better by Tuesday, we will try a different treatment." The fact that the attack can be terminated rapidly by ECT should also be mentioned, if the patient is rational. Its existence as a longstop may improve morale, even if it is not necessary to use the treatment, but it is already the subject of much harmful misinformation. The Minnesota Multiphasic Personality Inventory (MMPI), skillfully interpreted, and any history of impulsive solutions to life crises, are important indices of suicide risk in the controlled, private, and uncommunicative patient. Most elderly patients who contemplate suicide seek professional help before making the attempt.

Anxiously depressed patients with weeping, hand wringing, and overt delusions of illness or guilt have the great advantage of obviousness: Their condition is usually correctly diagnosed. Retarded and undemonstrative patients run a greater risk: Their illness may be mistaken for "dementia," and their suicidal potential, particularly when domiciliary treatment with tricyclics begins to work, may be underrated. The indices of depression must be inquired for, especially in quiet older patients, whose frequent and uncharacteristic visits to the doctor with minor complaints may cover a depressive conviction that they have a fatal illness.

Mania may not only alternate with depression but also be "mixed" with it, in patients who are simultaneously aggressive, depressed, hyperactive rather than akinetic, and dysphoric. This mixture, rather than the elated mania seen in some younger patients, is probably most common in the old. Whereas the younger housewife may begin spring cleaning at three in the morning as a manifestation of unusual and uncontrollable energy, the older person may do so out of fear and anxiety, but both are manic. In very old people with major physical illness, mania is almost always mistaken for senile ill temper.

The main diagnostic hazards are failure to notice treatable affective disorder altogether, so that the patient's misery is prolonged or suicide occurs; mistaking agitated depression with delusions (e.g., that the patient is being poisoned or is damned) and hallucinations (that voices accuse them of sodomy or murder) for schizophrenia; confusing apathetic depression with brain damage, which may coexist in some cases; and overlooking drug toxicity.

The treatment of depression must in all cases be active, because it is a controllable, life-threatening illness. "Where there is depression, there is hope." Psychotherapy is persuasive and supportive. The main requirements are concern and time; it should not be historical or argumentative. Medication should be begun with tricyclics, which work best where anorexia, insomnia, retardation, and fatigue are present and the onset is insidious. The side effects are immediate, and may be hazardous in the old, but they decline with time, and a therapeutic effect should be seen within five days to three weeks. A dangerous period in agitated and potentially suicidal patients is the interval before the drug begins to improve mood, when side effects are maximal and the patient gets tired of waiting to feel better. At this stage, the first evidence of improving activity may be a suicide attempt. Old persons should be started on approximately one-third the normal adult dose with monitored increase, a process which may lengthen the waiting period. With amitryptilene or doxepin, 25 mg are given initially; dosage should rise to 150 mg by 25-mg increments every five days. Less anticholinergic drugs (imipramine, desipramine) may be given in divided doses; more anticholinergic or more sedative tricyclics, in a single bolus at night. Anticholinergic effects on attendant conditions (prostatic enlargement, glaucoma), and cardiotoxicity should be guarded against. All tricyclics have a quinidine-like action on rhythmicity; doxepin has reputedly the least overdose and cardiotoxic potential (see Table 3.1).

If tricyclics are ineffective, especially in so-called atypical depression associated with obsessions, or where there is a past history of depression associated with migraine cycles, depersonalization, déjà pensé, and dream scintillations (Forbes, 1949; Saul, 1965), MAOIs should not be withheld. American teaching regarding these drugs is alarmist in tone. The fact that they require dietary restrictions and limit the possibility of emergency interventions by cross-reacting with drugs, anesthetics, and analgesics should be offset against the transformation they can produce in chronically disabled patients. Isocarboxazid or phenelzine should be tried before tranylcypromine. In geriatric patients, it would obviously be prudent to begin tranylcypromine administration in hospital. When a patient who responds well is discharged on maintenance doses (phenelzine, 15 or 30mg/day, with instructions to increase the dose to 1 mg/kg body weight/day at the first sign of recurrence), hypotension is a more threatening and more common complication than hypertensive crisis. A few patients may lose intractable or lifelong recurrent depression on a combination of phenelzine with a tricyclic (Shuckit et al., 1971; Ponto et al., 1977): This combination should be administered only in a psychiatric unit. Sustained mood improvement with MAOIs correlates strongly, at the outset of treatment, with suppression of REM sleep, a process which takes seven to nine days (Dunleavy and Oswald, 1973). The symptom constellation which responds best to MAOIs includes hypochondriasis, somatic anxiety, irritability, phobias, and anergia, the attributes of so-called atypical depression (Tyrer, 1976). The degree of response depends largely on biochemical idiosyncrasy, chiefly speed of acetylation (Johnstone and Marsh, 1973; Quitkin et al., 1979). Guilt, delusions, intense depressive mood, ideas of reference, nihilistic ideas, and, in general, the stigmata of severe typical depression indicate a poor response potential and suggest treatment with ECT and long-term lithium if distress is not relieved by tricyclics.

The pharmacology of phenelzine has been reviewed by Robinson et al. (1978). Emphasis here on MAOIs as an adjuvant in geriatric practice, for the treatment of non-endogenous depression and phobic disorders with or without somatization, is justified by the reluctance, until recently, among American psychiatrists to use them. European practice, however, bears out their value if employed with reasonable prudence. In Bethune et al.'s (1964) study, the incidence of toxic effects was 8.4% prior to the recognition of food factors in hypertensive crisis. With dietary precautions, major side effects are rare (Raskin, 1972). Toxicity in the elderly, given reasonable precautions, is in fact usually less for MAOIs, hypotension aside, than for tricyclics, because there is no anticholinergic blockade. Senile confusion and memory loss are themselves symptoms of defective cholinergic transmission. Apart from arrhythmias, tachycardia, urinary retention, other physical effects, which can aggravate depression and threaten vital processes, and severe discomfort (dry mouth, dizziness), tricyclics can induce confusion severe enough to require physostigmin, which itself is hazardous to the old. The only common mental side effect of MAOIs is an increased tendency for depression to pass through a manic stage during recovery. A nontoxic MAOI which could be displaced from gut-cell MAO by tyramine is a geriatric drug devoutly to be wished for. In contrast to those of MAOIs, maintenance doses of tricyclics usually must be substantial, but because of the suicide risk, large amounts of either type of drug should not be prescribed (not more than, say, 1.5 gm for tricyclics or one week's supply of phenelzine) until stability has been observed over several months. Suicidal poisoning with tricyclics is exceptionally lethal.

Although some late-life depressions are truly refractory, it is important not to arrive at this conclusion, or to persist in it, simply on the grounds that at some time, a tricyclic antidepressant has failed to improve mood. Tricyclics cannot be said to have failed unless (a) adequate time, up to three weeks at full doses, has been allowed for each drug prescribed; (b) blood levels have been checked—an expensive and still not widely available investigation which is essential in refractory late-life depression; and (c) both stimulant and sedative antidepressant tricyclics have been tried.

Blood levels must be established, because tolerance may decline rapidly with age. In some patients with a record of response to these drugs during previous attacks, dose has been increased on the usual schedule with marked exacerbation of symptoms, especially confusion, and blood levels then show gross overdose, even in the absence of atropine-like peripheral effects (Appelbaum et al., 1979). With reduced dose and blood-level monitoring, a good remission may occur. Both classes of tricyclic drugs must be adequately tried. The widespread view that "tricyclic antidepressants are interchangeable" is possibly correct in bulk but not in detail. Where depressions respond easily, it may be true. But the stimulant (protryptilene, desipramine, imipramine) and the sedative, tertiary amine group (doxepin, amitryptilene) probably affect different amine pumps—those for norepinephrine and serotonin, respectively (Maas, 1975). These correspond to "fight" and "freeze" reaction states of animals in the face of stress: Imipramine apparently affects both mechanisms. Since the specific chemistry of individual depressive cases is still unclear, and individual patients often show anergy, agitation, or both at different times, at least one drug from each group must be tried successively before tricyclics are said to have failed. Clinical impressions may determine which is to be tried first, but they have failed in double-blind trials to predict drug response (Schildkraut et al., 1973). Moreover, even if both groups eventually have antidepressant effects, norepinephrinergic drugs often make lethargic patients feel better and serotoninergic drugs make them feel worse in the short term, and vice versa in agitated patients. These short-term "side effects" have an important impact on morale and compliance during the waiting period before the major antidepressant effects develop: The patient's assessment of the drug should accordingly be noted, not dismissed as part of a depressed attitude. In depressed, confused, and lethargic people who are negativistic, the experience which they are undergoing depends on their inability to muster mental resources. They may show mechanically expressed agitation (reiterating "No," or "It's terrible" in a perseverative manner), but the clinician will recognize lethargy as predominant. In such cases, protryptilene with or without small doses of methylphenidate is more likely to work than a sedative tricyclic. Agitated patients can be pushed into toxic confusion by an added phenothiazine if tolerance is low, as it often is in old age: Phenothiazines inhibit the metabolism of most tricyclic drugs and raise blood levels. In geriatric practice, cardiotoxicity or other hazards may limit the choice of a drug, but every unresponsive case must be reviewed by a psychopharmacologist in order to avoid further depressing the patient by a series of treatment failures. Sleep pattern studies, MHPG excretion levels (Beckmann and Goodwin, 1975), and response to a test dose of an amphetamine may eventually offer a better guide to the type of chemical deficit and the drug of first choice (Schildkraut et al., 1973). (MHPG (3-methoxy-4-hydroxyphenyl glycol) is a metabolite of norepinephrine and a measure of its turnover.)

In intense depression with florid psychotic symptoms, pressure toward suicide, or great misery, especially if unaccompanied by lethargy, tricyclics cannot offer speedy relief, MAOIs are typically ineffective, and early resort to ECT, regardless of age, is a humane procedure, comparable with the emergency relief of severe physical pain. As in all depressive conditions, it is necessary to view the illness as a life-threatening emergency, which it is. Full-thickness ECT can produce confusion and usually produces amnesia. In elderly patients, these effects may be exaggerated, but permanent intellectual deficits after ECT usually represent preexistent organicity which was masked by the depression, not results of the treatment. If organicity is known to coexist, unilateral ECT to the nondominant hemisphere, although less effective, is also less apt to produce confusion (Hall, 1974). In most cases, the patient, even if temporarily confused, feels so much better with the lifting of the depression that intellectual function improves. Although tricyclics lower the seizure threshold, therapy can be planned so that the improvement following ECT covers the lag period before their effects on mood become evident. The contraindications for ECT in the elderly are probably identical with those for dental extraction under general anesthesia, with the reservation that the risk of treatment is commonly less than that of suicide, and certainly less than that of prolonged severe illness, if treatment is not undertaken. This equation should be presented to relatives, patients, or professional colleagues intimidated by propaganda against the use of judicious and indicated ECT on the European model.

In planning the use of ECT in geriatric patients, it is important to remember that recovery time after unilateral treatment is increased fivefold and after bilateral treatment ninefold in patients over 65 (Fraser and Glass, 1978) and there is far greater sensitivity than in the young to cumulation and to interval effects.

"Modern ECT is an atraumatic procedure administered under general anesthesia with full oxygenation and muscle relaxation. It is safe and effective, and in properly selected patients it produces highly predictable therapeutic results which are unequalled by any other treatment method" (Abrams, 1979). This is no less true in geriatric practice.

Lithium is the most effective agent available for the prevention of recurrent affective disorder (Coppen et al., 1978)—more so in mania than in depression, but deserving of a trial in either. In mania, it is more effective, although less rapid in action, than haloperidol. It is effective in older patients (Foster et al., 1977), but careful monitoring of blood concentrations is required because of the rapidity with which electrolyte disturbances can appear in the old, and the possibility of arrhythmias. The method of taking an initial series of blood readings, pushing lithium dosage until tremor just appears, and then slightly reducing the dose is not reliable in the geriatric age group and may be hazardous. The effective blood level is between 0.6 and 1.5 meq/liter (Salkind, 1970; Fry and Marks, 1971). Heart failure, renal failure, and conditions likely to disturb sodium balance, including medication with diuretics, are contraindications. Suicide attempts with lithium can produce permanent brain damage, including seizure disorders.

The relief and prevention of recurrent mania are by now a familiar indication for lithium. In Coppen et al.'s (1971) classical study of bipolar and unipolar affective illness, including unipolar depressions, 86% of treated patients were rated symptom free during treatment as opposed to 8% of the placebo group, and only 11% of the lithium group were rated unchanged or worse. In view of its relatively low toxicity, and its compatibility with other antidepressants, trial of lithium is accordingly worthwhile (a) in any recurrent affective disorder, even if the cycle is irregular, and (b) in any psychosis which appears to have an affective component, since many supposed schizophrenics with affective symptoms are responsive, if gross contraindications are absent.

There is, finally, a group of last-resort drugs which occasionally relieve depression, or appear to do so. Their usefulness in geriatric medicine, or in psychiatry generally, has not been documented, but they can be borne in mind. Thyroid extract (Evans, 1970) and low-dose androgens are such drugs. Thyroid supplements can increase the efficacy of tricyclic drugs. In cases of extreme anergia in old people with few truly depressive symptoms, or where anticholinergic antidepressants are not tolerated, methylphenidate alone (Kaplitz, 1975), starting with homeopathic doses, occasionally produces striking benefit. Forced increase in weight by a regimen of porridge and small doses of insulin will occasionally terminate a long-lasting, low-grade depression with marked weight loss. Some lifelong intractable depressive cycles are migrainous; others are associated with occult convulsive disorder. The former often respond dramatically to MAOIs, the latter to carbamazepine (Helleckson et al., 1979). L-tryptophan is another experimental agent which has some record of success (Coppen et al., 1967). It is compatible with MAOIs and tricyclics and is apparently an effective hypnotic.

Little work has been done to study such accessory drugs specifically in geriatrics. Salzman (Salzman and Shader, 1975) found that methylphenidate was an effective antidepressant and improved memory in females but not in males, who did better on mild sedatives: Diazepam was particularly likely to cause confusion in women, less so in men. This type of finding, even when statistical, must be viewed in the light of the protean character of "depression" and "memory deficit" in the old—in other words, in terms of case selection— but sex differences may indeed exist and should be further documented. At all ages, depressions can be self-limiting (so that medication may take undue credit). They are also extremely prone to recurrence, especially in the old. Medication must be planned so that it can be maintained over years on a precautionary basis; this can be done with small doses, particularly of MAOIs, with quick increase at the first sign of trouble.

Finally, not only may depression aggravate dementia, but dementias may present as depression. Of a series of insidious-onset presenile dementias, 50% were initially diagnosed as affective disorder (Liston, 1977). In some cases where depression of late onset fails to respond to treatment, underlying Alzheimerism may be present. The fact that dementia can be convincingly imitated by tricyclic overdosage makes blood-level monitoring particularly necessary if a dementing change is suspected.

SCHIZOPHRENIA

The geriatric psychiatrist encounters schizophrenia in three ways: He may be called to deal with the patient who has grown old in psychotic illness; he may be required to investigate "late paraphrenia"; and he may be able, by correct diagnosis, to salvage the declining years of some of those patients in whom the gross overuse of "schizophrenia" as a diagnostic label has caused schizoaffective illness to be missed. The last of these categories may well be the most important, since schizoaffective illness responds, sometimes dramatically, to correct treatment, however long the history.

Schizophrenia is a constitutional, and, once manifest, usually a lifelong condition, which can be palliated by antipsychotics and supportive therapy, but not as a rule removed (Harrow et al., 1978). In some people, the degree of disturbance is minor and compatible with social adjustment during much of their life, but with the pressures and infirmities of age, the adjustment may fail (and relatives become more willing to admit that the patient is more than eccentric). These cases are among those which present as late paraphrenia. When mental illness appears at any age with Schneider's (1959) "first-rank symptoms" (ideas of influence, hearing thoughts spoken aloud, transference of thoughts by and to others, somatic hallucinations, delusions), the diagnosis of schizophrenia still requires, negatively, the exclusion of toxic and similar organic causes, and, positively, a history indicating that any mental illness in relatives should itself have been schizophrenic and not affective, the absence of affective components, the absence of complete remission, even between attacks, and where any of the forgoing conditions are unfulfilled, an unsuccessful therapeutic trial of tricyclics, lithium, and MAOIs. The evidence for such a judgment cannot be available in a first attack, but by the geriatric age, it is almost bound to be available if sought.

This view of schizophrenia as a diagnostic entity runs counter to Bleuler's (1972) lifetime study of patients so diagnosed, which indicated that they often experienced remission or made good adjustment, so that deterioration after the first few years was rare. It has to be borne in mind, however, that his account of the natural history of the disease presumes the old and traditional diagnostic criteria, which included a category of "good prognosis schizophrenia" now in serious doubt. There probably is indeed a category of patients who are schizophrenic by the criteria of family history and nonresponse to antidepressants and whose illness remits, or is extremely mild, until they are overtaken in the geriatric period by a combination of socioenvironmental stress, attack on ego defenses, and age changes in brain catecholamine metabolism, and who then either develop recrudescent psychosis or are diagnosed as psychotic for the first time. These are the "late paraphrenics" who figure in geropsychiatric literature. Roth and Morrissey (1952) found only about 10% of such cases in the psychiatric hospital intake. Because schizophrenia itself almost certainly represents a specific neurochemical disorder, or a neurochemical idiosyncrasy with a structural basis, there is no a priori reason why a first attack should not occur late in life, especially as other disorders affecting neurotransmission become more common at that time.

A first attack of psychotic symptoms in youth or middle life is always difficult to diagnose correctly. There are undoubtedly patients who have only one such attack and who recover completely. Slavish obedience by the diagnostician to the dogma of "first rank symptoms" led to the creation of a category of "good prognosis schizophrenia" which probably concealed the existence of a number of disorders with differing natural histories, including schizoaffective illness, "hysterical" psychosis (Cavenar et al., 1979; Spiegel and Fink 1979), and acute episodic psychosis.

The geriatrician's task is easier in that the complete record may be available, but more difficult in that facts about past illnesses may be hard to get. Patient, relatives, and physician may all have been influenced by past diagnoses: A family mythology, either of resignation or of denial, may have grown up around the patient's mental illness, and the patient may have had many years of appropriate or inappropriate psychotropic medication. A patient who had the misfortune of becoming ill during the heyday of schizophrenia as a catch-all in American psychiatry will have been under strong pressure to fulfill the diagnostician's expectations. Accordingly, in dealing with longstanding illness, the geriatrician must (a) consider the present mental problem in all its aspects, (b) review the history with allowances made for the fact that the original diagnosis, with which patients and relatives have lived, may have been made 50 years ago, and (c) reconsider the diagnosis in the light of the most recent psychiatric knowledge.

All the first-rank symptoms of "schizophrenia" as it has been commonly diagnosed may occur, and do occur frequently, in so-called schizoaffective illness and in manic-depressive psychosis (MDP) (Pope and Lipinski, 1978), especially during atypical manias when feelings of passivity predominate over hyperactivity. The incidence of first-rank symptoms in MDP has run as high as 70% in some hospital series (Carlson and Goodwin, 1973). Correction of the diagnosis, and trial of lithium in particular where it has not been tried, is a major task of geriatric psychiatry after a period of medical fashion during which schizophrenia has been grossly overdiagnosed, under the influence of the maxim that "even a trace of schizophrenia is schizophrenia" (Lewis and Piotrowsky, 1954) coupled with some equally erroneous, although different, psychoanalytic uses of the term. If the patient, however long the history, (a) shows affective features; (b) has any relative with frank MDP, or with a record of suicide, alcoholism, or episodes of excitement; (c) has had any clear periods (best judged by occupational record) between episodes of illness when no thought disorder was evident; (d) has never been given a trial of lithium, or (e) has been diagnosed in the past as suffering from "good prognosis schizophrenia;" the provisional assumption should be made that, first-rank symptoms notwithstanding, this is not schizophrenia. Aggressive therapy should be begun with lithium and antidepressants, on the basis that even a trace of affective disorder is likely to be affective disorder, even if phenothiazines are also given to reduce bizarre behavior. In the early stages of these cases, the presence of affective elements; the evidence of depression or mood changes in the family history, if they were present; and, usually, the lack of the typical and ominous "praecox feeling" engendered in the physician who attempts, and fails, to make contact with the patient at interview, and which accompanies flatness or incongruity of affect, might have given the clue. By the time later life is reached, family history may be inaccessible, and flattening of affect accompanied by oddity of response may be a natural consequence of a life spent in and out of institutions on heavy medication. Positive evidence of affective problems in relatives and a story of genuine remission in an exacting occupation are probably the two most important review items. If there is doubt, a trial of lithium is indicated. High scores on the MMPI 6, 8 and "F" ("meshuggeneh") scales, merely indicate that first-rank symptoms were present. High scores on the affective scales should lead to an immediate review of the diagnosis of schizophrenia. The leading consideration, at this late stage of presentation, is whether a change of diagnosis might not substitute a controllable for a suppressible illness. Moreover, although long-term antipsychotic therapy can produce serious symptoms, neither lithium nor the antidepressants when properly administered will usually make schizophrenic symptoms, if genuine, permanently worse. Tricyclics may aggravate illness, but the results can be speedily controlled with antipsychotics and withdrawal of the antidepressant. Even where the picture is complicated in old patients by brain damage, response to correct therapy can still occur if the disorder is affective. In these, as in other geriatric cases, the physician learns that neither the size of the dossier nor the unanimity of previous opinions should preclude a revision of old diagnoses.

In the presence of severe thought disorder and disabling hallucinations and delusions, there is no present alternative to antipsychotic drugs. Their use in the old is beset by side effects. Tardive dyskinesia is most often in the prescriber's mind, because many elderly people seem to be on the verge of an idiopathic syndrome very like it: Lip pursing and minor Parkinsonian symptoms increase with age even in the absence of frank Parkinsonism. It is equally possible to substitute for the distress of mental illness the equally taxing distress of akathisia (Raskin, 1972; van Putten, 1975). On the other hand, some patients, especially those in whom paranoia is the only socially disabling symptom, respond well and are relieved. Whether phenothiazines, haloperidol, or thiothixenes are used, the initial dose should be small, and increments should be made no more than every seven days (which is about the length of time necessary for untoward side effects to develop) unless a genuine emergency exists. Very small doses of phenothiazines are sufficient to control intermittent (usually evening) symptoms, the so-called sundown syndrome. Butyrophenones and thiothixene are less apt to produce orthostatic hypotension but are more apt to produce akathisia than phenothiazines.

If thought disorder is minor and anxiety great, doxepin or amitriptilene, or a sedative benzodiazepin (chlorazepate, prazepam) in low initial doses is sometimes enough (although in these cases, the diagnosis of schizophrenia is called in question by the large affective element). Long-term dosage with several assorted drugs, or with the "minor" tranquilizers, has no place in geriatrics. Some schizophrenics unresponsive to other drugs have been reported to benefit from a trial of propranolol (Yorkston et al., 1977), but these were chiefly younger patients with bizarre thought content. Propranolol appears to act specifically on the orienting reflex (the response to unfamiliarity); thus its effectiveness in panic states, which in the old are rarely of schizophrenic origin.

Hallucinosis and paranoia following cataract surgery are transient: They appear to be a specific result of the operation, not merely a response to sensory deprivation (Summers and Reich, 1979).

Paranoid symptoms are not diagnostic of schizophrenia (Manschreck and Petri, 1978). They occur in up to 40% of psychiatric unit admissions and are equally common or more common in general-practice psychiatry. There is no single condition of which they are diagnostic, being seen in affective disorder, especially when a depressed patient believes that others share his self-condemnation; in organic brain syndrome, often as part of a defense or coping mechanism; and in suspicious individuals who are not psychotic. These patients often have ideas of reference: People may be interfering with their property, eyeing them in a significant manner, or mustering an elaborate conspiracy against them. Psychotic patients may also hear derogatory voices accusing them of sexual irregularity or discussing their behavior (see Tables 3.2 and 3.3).

The importance of recognizing this nonspecificity is that while in the short-term almost all paranoid ideation is reduced in intensity by phenothiazines, paranoia in affective illness responds in the long term to lithium or antidepressants. In many cases, properly interpreted psychometric tests (MMPI, Holzmann inkblot test) will discriminate between affective and schizophrenic paranoia, however bizarre the patient's behavior (Freedman and Schwab, 1978). In geriatric patients, organic brain syndrome must also be excluded; where it is psychotic in manifestation, about 63% of patients will show paranoid features. Old, anxious, and confused people who are sick but not demented may show transient paranoid episodes which express exasperation rather than thought disorder and which subside with supportive mea-

TABLE 3.2. Diagnoses of Paranoid and Nonparanoid Patients

Diagnostic category (DSM II)	No. of patients	% Paranoid
Organic brain syndromes		
Psychotic	19	63
Nonpsychotic	6	0
Psychoses		
Schizophrenia	81	68
Major affective disorders	36	50
Paranoid states	4	100
Other psychoses [a]	10	70
Neuroses	43	10
Personality disorders	37	12
Transient situation disturbances, other	28	3

[a] Psychotic depressive reactions.

From Freedman, R. and Schwab, P.J. (1978).

TABLE 3.3. "Nonpsychiatric" Causes of Paranoid Symptoms

CNS
Temporal lobe epilepsy
Multiple sclerosis
Huntington's chorea
Presenile organic dementias

MEDICAL
Hypertensive encephalopathy
Pituitary and temporal lobe tumors
Postencephalitic Parkinsonism
Subdural hematoma
Subarachnoid hemorrhage
Fat embolism
Menzel's ataxia
Roussy–Levy syndrome
Motor neurone disease
Muscular dystrophies
Narcolepsy
Delirium of all causes

METABOLIC
Uremia
Wilson's disease
Systemic lupus erythematosus
Acute intermittent porphyria
B12 deficiency
Hepatic failure
Portacaval shunt
Hemodialysis
Hypoglycemia
Carboxyhemoglobinemia

CHROMOSOMAL ABNORMALITY
Klinefelter's syndrome
Turner's syndrome
47XYY

ENDOCRINE
Addison's disease
Cushing's syndrome
Hypopituitarism
Hyperthyroidism, myxedema

INFECTIONS
Syphilis
Malaria
Encephalitis lethargica
Typhus
Trypanosomiasis

DRUGS
Alcohol
Marijuana
Amphetamines
Bromides
Barbiturates
Cocaine
N2O
Withdrawal psychoses

THERAPEUTIC AGENTS
Amphetamines
Pentazocin
ACTH and cortisone
L-Dopa
Methyldopa–haloperidol
Methyltestosterone–imipramine
Anticholinergic agents
Phenytoin

Adapted from Manschreck, T. (1979).

sures, including, as a rule, rescue from the family or other situation which precipitated them. One striking form of paranoia which can occur in old as well as younger patients is unfounded pathological jealousy. In old men whose sense of self-value is eroded by age or the threat of dependency, this form of jealousy—often wildly inappropriate—may dramatize their sense of loss, but the fact that it may also appear intelligible should not mislead the physician, because violence may result. The patient should be admitted to hospital rather than counseled in the office. Phenothiazines or haloperidol usually reduce the importance and hostility of the jealous feelings, but full evaluation is necessary before such a patient is discharged, or mischief may result, especially if the partner is frail and the couple lives alone. Alcohol may produce a return of hostile behavior even after the acute disturbance subsides. In some seemingly unlikely instances, the "paranoid" suspicion turns out to be true, despite the venerable age of the parties. There is often an overtly sexual problem in addition to any symbolic "loss of virility" connected with the aging process. In one case which came to our attention, inability of the surgeon to explain in plain language post-prostatectomy ejaculatory changes to a prospective patient played a part in setting the scene for jealous paranoia.

At the age of 81, Mr. G. formed the opinion that his 73-year-old wife was pursuing a liaison with a neighbor to whom she had been introduced at a seniors club by "two old yentas." Mr. G. set traps for her, ostensibly going to town and returning to find her still in her nightgown. Finally he confronted her, suggested a divorce, and in the course of the ensuing argument threatened to kill all three of them. To frighten her into good behavior he went, accompanied by his wife, to purchase a pistol. Instead he frightened himself, for his son and daughter-in-law had him summarily removed to hospital.

Mr. G. was a vigorous, amusing, and verbal man. His story carried conviction, but his hostility was fading with reflection. His wife was an alert, attractive, and managing lady, but affectionate toward him. At consultation rounds after a private talk with the patient, the physician was unexpectedly confronted by husband, wife, son, and the ward team. In these circumstances it was necessary to de-emphasize the facts at issue and get them all out of the room as fast as possible, in order to avoid playing Solomon, attacking either the patient's sanity or the family's veracity.

Mr. G.'s troubles actually started seven years previously, when a suprapubic prostatectomy had been performed. Neither spouse had been made aware of the sexual implications beyond an embarrassed remark by the surgeon to Mrs. G. that she must understand that she would bear no more children. Since she was then 66, this seem self-evident. After surgery, Mr. G. found himself potent but unable to ejaculate, which deeply depressed him. His potency soon declined and he blamed his wife for permitting the operation. She in turn became "so busy she had no time to fret," whereas he "had nothing to do." Mr. G. bitterly regretted his lost ejaculatory capacity and his wife's philosophical response to it, projecting his feelings on her: Women have no need for ejaculation or erection, he said, and their sexuality outlasts that of men.

Our impression was that having been displaced psychologically as head of the household, Mr. G. had "staged a hanging" and might now have made his point. Couple counseling was arranged, with small doses of thiothixene, so as not to aggravate his potency problems. It was deemed important that his dramatic com-mital should not become a weapon in future family strife. Unfortunately, when he was allowed home on leave, he harrassed and attempted to throttle his wife. The symptoms subsided on full doses of haloperidol, but it was judged better that they should live apart for a few weeks until the emotional "relevance" of the delusion faded. In about six weeks he returned home on minimal medication. Mr. G.'s paranoia clearly dramatized the mortification of a man who, in his own words, "did not kvetch a lot," and was the climax of a long interpersonal struggle. Whether it could have been avoided by proper preoperative counseling is not clear.

A year later, the paranoria had faded and had been replaced by ingravescent cognitive and memory loss.

Paranoid schizophrenia may be a distinct disorder; its age of onset is later than that of other forms (mean, 42.0 years). Genetic evidence is conflicting, but fewer paranoid schizophrenics may have schizophrenic relatives than those with early-onset forms. Persecutory delusions are more prominent than thought disorder, emotional incongruity, or catatonic states, and paranoid illness, even when diagnosed as schizophrenic, has a better prognosis and a higher compatibility with job stability than other forms. These distinctions simply mean that its nosological status is unclear: The diagnosis would imply a frankly psychotic illness with many paranoid features and some first-rank symptoms of schizophrenia which failed to improve on antidepressants. The diagnosis should be made rarely in view of the stigma of a finding of "schizophrenia" on the patient. Therapy apart, labels in paranoia have a prognostic implication, because neither late paraphrenia nor "paranoid schizophrenia" in the elderly shortens life. By contrast, where similar symptoms have a basis in early organic dementia, physical and mental health usually deteriorate rapidly. Apart from this, the distinction between "late paraphrenia" with paranoid features (in older persons, usually with multiple sensory defects, and a record of previous eccentricity) and "paranoid schizophrenia" (in older persons without previous mental illness until late adulthood) is an academic exercise of less practical importance than the recognition of paranoias occurring in affective illness or as the presenting symptom of neurological disorder, drug effects, uremia, intermittent porphyria, and a number of other conditions calling for diagnosis and treatment, which are increasingly overlooked in the mentally sick and difficult old. The sensory-defect contribution to paranoia, its almost total nonspecificity as a symptom, and the prejudice latent in a long textbook association of the syndrome with "senility" and with schizophrenia should constantly be borne in mind. Paranoia can be produced in some subjects by a wide range of drugs with anticholinergic side effects, including tricyclic antidepressants themselves.

THE MUTE PATIENT: DEPRESSED, DEMENTED, PSYCHOTIC, OR ANGRY?

The incidence of mutism in patients reaching a geriatric psychiatry unit is higher than among the young. It can be a confusing symptom. Leaving aside the aphasias and akinetic mutism following stroke, the physician has to determine, like the old-time British jury, whether the patient is "mute of malice" (i.e., not talking) or mute by act of God (unable to talk). The patient may say nothing, respond by minimal phonation or gesture but clearly understand what is said and obey instructions, or reply monosyllabically ("Can you tell me your name?" "Yes"). The problem is to ascertain what the mute one is experiencing. The poverty of response can indicate depression, anger and regression, intense preoccupation with confusing inner experiences such as hallucinations, intense lethargy, or dementia to the point at which, although questions are understood, the sufferer mistrusts his or her ability to reply coherently. Mutism can be a "last straw" response in unremitting illness, especially depression, when the patient has suffered much from many physicians and anger combines with despair. Thus a 60-year-old man whose most recent depressive attack had resisted ECT, tricyclics, and MAOIs, passed from monosyllabic preoccupation to total mutism, responding only by intention movements, but obeyed all instructions accurately, spoke occasionally on the ward, and more frequently to his wife, with whom he played Scrabble. He also volunteered the name of the winning team in a major football match.

Where mutism accompanies soft neurological signs and dementia, it can, if not vascular, reflect the frontal abulia of Pick's disease, more often than the global function loss of other dementias. Deep psychotic preoccupation often responds to haloperidol. In voluntary mutism with retention of faculties, it can be worth trying to elicit response under amytal to ascertain what the patient is thinking.

True catatonic mutism is not very common in the senium: When it occurs, it pays to recall that catatonia, as Kahlbaum first pointed out in 1874, is far more often a depressive equivalent than a manifestation of schizophrenia. Its termination by ECT commonly unveils a manic depressive psychosis, although it may also occur in dementias, and it is an entirely nonspecific manifestation (Abrams and Taylor, 1976). In unexplained catatonia, trial of naloxone would be theoretically justified.

4

ORGANIC
DEMENTING PROCESSES

Old age is not a cause of dementia. The dementias which accumulate with age, once secondary confusional and pseudodemented states have been excluded, have an extensive and varied pathology (Seltzer and Sherwin, 1978; see Table 4.1). In subdividing the diagnosis of "organic brain syndrome," once it is established that organicity exists, all of these possibilities must be excluded, but only three are really common: atrophic brain syndrome (Alzheimer's disease, senile type), multiple infarctive dementia ("cerebral atherosclerosis"), and chronic alcohol poisoning (which may present as a typical Korsakoff psychosis, but often does not). In view of the prevalence of alcohol abuse, it is difficult to know whether it is a determinant in the preceding two pathologies, but additional alcohol damage is often probably present, and dementia may follow one episode of heavy drinking in a patient whose brain is already compromised.

Differential diagnosis is important, because although all three types of dementia improve with humane treatment and conservation of declining capacity, some cases of embolic dementia can be strikingly improved by medication. Obvious neurological signs are not prominent in Alzheimerism: They can be prominent in embolic processes and in Pick's dementia, but Pick's dementia (resembling Alzheimer but without plaques and tangles) is rare. Another "presenile dementia" of great importance in spite of its uncommonness is Jakob—Creutzfeldt disease, because this is due to a slow virus, is transmissible to healthy persons, for example, by instruments, and presents a hazard to staff if missed (Gajdusek et al., 1977). Myoclonus is an important sign.

Many authors of textbooks and teachers have suggested that aggressive diagnostic efforts in late-life dementia are a waste of time and money. A more correct view would be that the diagnosis and investigation of dementia exactly parallel the diagnosis and investigation of malignancy. In both instances, a high proportion of cases will prove to be too advanced for rescue. In both instances, support and palliation are possible. In both instances, the cost-accountancy aspects of exhaustive investigation are overridden by the possibility of effectual cure in a proportion of cases if the nature of the disease is established early enough. Both cancers and dementias are responsible for enormous personal and social costs—the second possibly greater in dementias because of their chronicity and their requirement of prolonged bed occupancy. The attitude of medical impotence and "giving up" in the face of a diagnosis of dementia (Ernst et al., 1977) had its parallel in older attitudes to malignancy, when curable or helpable patients or those with misdiagnosed nonmalignant conditions were permitted to die through benign neglect. Aside from any active therapy of major dementing processes, about 15% of all those presenting with "senile dementia" have correctable disorders (Wells, 1978). Many drugs appear to improve the quality of life or delay deterioration in true dementias (cyclandelate, hydergine, coumadin, and others have been favorably reported), provided the condition is recognized and attacked early: The results here are roughly comparable with those in the early days of cancer chemotherapy, in that no medication will restore the fully deteriorated patient. For these reasons, early diagnosis and active differential diagnosis are of the greatest importance. The analogy with cancer may serve to impress the point upon students, who indicate the social convention by responding quite differently to the two conditions.

Organic dementing processes may be caused by a wide range of pathologies, from congenital disorders to tumors. Fortunately, although these causes do produce slight differences in the natural history and presentation, and in most cases neurological signs, they are mostly seen by the neurologist, not the geriatrician. The geriatrician's concern is substantially with four topics only: the three common dementing diseases of old age—Alzheimerism, infarctive dementia, and alcohol syndrome—and with the exclusion of all other causes of dementia, including those that are treatable by treatment of the underlying disease.

Alzheimer-type changes account for about 50% of senile-type dementias in hospital patients, infarctive changes for about 15%, and a further 20% show both (Corsellis, 1962; Roth, 1971). Of the remaining 15% with other pathologies, a fair number will be due to alcohol damage and others to intractable diseases. In office patients, the proportion of treatable—reversible dementing processes is higher because of the presence of pseudodementias (depression, symptomatic confusion, medication effects). Once these are excluded and dementia established, the mission becomes one of vigilance for the treatable case. This is a major task of the geriatric psychiatric assessment unit. Tables 4.1–4.5 give an excellent picture of the practicalities of the undertaking. Recognition of the atypical, and possibly treatable, "senile dementia" rests heavily on clinical alertness to unusual features (associated

TABLE 4.1.   The Causes of Progressive Dementia

Primary cerebral degenerations	Intracranial mass lesions
Alzheimer's disease and senile dementia	Tumor
Multiinfarct dementia	Subdural hematomas
Pick's disease	Hydrocephalus
Huntington's chorea	Obstructive
Jakob–Creutzfeldt disease	Communicating
Disseminated sclerosis	Secondary to systemic disease
Spinocerebellar degenerations	Hypothyroidism
Wilson's disease	Hypocalcemia
Parkinsonism and its variants	Hypoglycemia
Punch-drunk syndrome	Porphyria
Cerebral infections and inflammations	Vitamin B_{12} deficiency
Neurosyphilis	Hepatic encephalopathy
Cranial arteritis	Renal dialysis
Disseminated lupus erythematosus	Malabsorption syndrome
Limbic encephalitis	Dementia in alcoholics
Multifocal leukoencephalopathy	

From Marsden, C. D. In Isaacs, A.D. and Post, F. (1978).

nonbrain symptoms, patchiness of intellectual deficit, presence of minimal neurological signs, absence of smooth and insidious progression).

With the availability of tomographic scanning, it becomes possible to visualize intracranial events in old people with symptoms of dementia. This is a patient group in whom the investigation is abundantly justified, given the excessive investment in such apparatus by American hospitals, but the object of the exercise is the exclusion of undiagnosed intracranial pathology and the search for the occasional, remediable cause, not the positive diagnosis of dementia. Although atrophic changes are confirmatory and suggestive, they unfortunately occur also in undemented subjects, so that the clinical condition and the results of serial psychometric tests must remain the chief agents of diagnosis. When Gosling (1955) investigated 68 obscure dementias in elderly patients by air encephalography, 15% had no radiographic evidence of at-

TABLE 4.2.   The Investigation of Dementia

Blood count and film	Chest X-ray
ESR	Skull X-ray
WR and serology	EEG
Thyroid function tests	Radioisotope brain scan
Electrolytes and urea, and liver function tests	EMI–CAT scan (or air encephalography)
Plasma calcium	CSF examination
Vitamin B_{12}	

From Marsden, C.D. In Isaacs, A.D. and Post, F. (1978).

TABLE 4.3. Outcome of Investigation of Dementia in Relation to Age at the Time of the Investigation

	Age (years)				
	50	50–59	60–69	70 +	Total
No. of patients	8	40	43	15	106
Not demented	5	10	5	2	22
Demented					
Intracranial space occupying mass	—	2	5	1	8
Multiinfarct dementia	—	1	5	2	8
Dementia in alcoholics	—	4	2	—	6
Possible normal pressure hydrocephalus	—	1	3	1	5
Jakob–Creutzfeldt disease	—	1	1	1	3
Huntington's chorea	2	1	—	—	3
Post-traumatic cerebral atrophy	—	1	—	—	1
Postsubarachnoid hemorrhage	1	—	—	—	1
Limbic encephalitis	—	—	1	—	1
Cerebral atrophy of unknown cause	—	19	21	8	48

From Marsden, C.D. In Isaacs, A.D. and Post, F. (1978).

rophy: At 5−10-year follow-up, of 49 of the patients showing atrophic changes, 16 were still living, none of whom was demented, and of these, most had been treated successfully for depression. Obvious atrophy in the presence of clinical dementia suggests organicity, but atrophy can occur in the undemented (Mann, 1973). Abnormal ventricular enlargement is not necessarily associated with dementia and may be absent in advanced brain disease (Van Boxel et al., 1978).

Tomography does, however, make serial noninvasive examination possible, although progressive radiological change is unlikely to occur without evidence of clinical deterioration. Cortical blood-isotope scanning may prove more useful in the future (Lassen et al., 1978), particularly in monitoring effects of therapy and identifying areas of silent infarction. Geriatric medicine is one area in which heavy investment in this type of sophisticated equipment may well prove necessary by the end of the century. Dementia in the absence of atrophy at computerized axial tomography (CAT) scan indicates re-evaluation for treatable illness (Fox et al., 1975). This and the detection of other pathologies are the main geriatric uses of CAT scans.

The longstanding distinction between "presenile" and "senile" forms of atrophic dementia is now no longer supportable, since the curve of incidence is continuous and shows no sign of bimodality (Heston and Mastri, 1977) and the two forms are genetically associated (Heston and Mastri, 1977; Sjogren et al., 1963). The symptom complex would best be referred to as Alzheimer's syndrome or Alzheimerism, analogous to Parkinsonism. It is characterized by progressive dementia focusing primarily on associative and recall processes, the absence of neurological localizing signs, the presence of characteristic plaques and tangles, and cortical atrophy—generalized, whereas that in Pick's

TABLE 4.4. Diagnoses in 80 "Organic Brain Syndrome" Patients

Diagnosis	Number
Presenile dementia	2
Senile dementia	19
And aphasia	1
And post-traumatic encephalopathy	1
And Korsakoff's syndrome (alcoholic)	1
Senile dementia supervening on schizophrenia	3
Multiinfarct dementia	1
Post-traumatic encephalopathy	3
Postanoxic encephalopathy	2
Postinfectious encephalopathy	
Herpes simplex encephalitis	1
Bacterial meningitis	1
Alcoholic dementia	10
And post-traumatic encephalopathy	3
And aphasia	1
And schizophrenia	1
Korsakoff's syndrome	
Alcohol and vitamin deficiency	7
Post-traumatic	1
Postanoxic	1
And schizophrenia	1
Aphasia	1
Multiple sclerosis	1
Schizophrenia	4
And history of prefrontal lobotomy	3
And Parkinson's disease (drug induced)	1
Schizophreniform psychosis with temporal lobe epilepsy	1
Affective psychosis (depression)	1
Mental retardation	1
Personality disorder (inadequate personality)	1
No apparent abnormality of the mental state	3
Undetermined	3

From Seltzer, B. and Sherwin, I. (1978).

disease is unilobar—due to massive selective loss of neurones (Bowen et al., 1977a,b), affecting chiefly cholinergic pathways.

In fact, the natural histories of Alzheimerism and of Parkinsonism are remarkably similar. Both appear to have genetic determinants (Martin et al., 1973), although not as marked as the genetic preferences of scrapie in sheep. If it were not for the recognition of the postencephalitic form, Parkinsonism could well have been regarded as a "senile" or self-explanatory process with a "presenile" form reflecting genetic bad luck. Indeed, plaques and tubular tangles indistinguishable from those of Alzheimer's disease occur in postencephalitic Parkinsonism, but in the nigral and cerulean neurones rather than in the hippocampus and cortex (Wisnewski et al., 1970). Parkinsonian dementia of Guam, in which rigidity and dementia occur usually without tremor,

TABLE 4.5. Number of Times Each Specific Diagnosis Was Made [a]

Diagnosis	Number
Senile dementia	22
Alcoholic dementia	15
Korsakoff's syndrome	11
Schizophrenia	10
Post-traumatic encephalopathy	7
Senile dementia supervening on schizophrenia	3
Aphasia	3
Presenile dementia	2
Postanoxic encephalopathy	2
Postinfectious encephalopathy	2
Multiinfarct dementia	1
Multiple sclerosis	1
Parkinson's disease	1
Schizophreniform psychosis with temporal lobe epilepsy	1
Affective psychosis	1
Mental retardation	1
Personality disorder	1

[a] The total is greater than 80 because some patients had two diagnoses.
From Seltzer, B. and Sherwin, I. (1978).

occupies a place intermediate between the other two classical syndromes but closer to the atypical, tremorless Parkinsonism of old age, which is eventually dementing in many cases. This disease, which causes about 7% of deaths among native Chamorro Guamese, appears to be well placed for an epidemiological attack like that mounted against kuru, but the small size of the population involved may obscure the fact that the cumulative incidence of Alzheimerism in older Americans is almost certainly the same or greater.

These similarities in natural history do not indicate that Alzheimerism and Parkinsonism are "one disease," although this may prove to be so (Hakim and Mathiason, 1978), or that either has a unitary etiology, but they suggest a common nosology in which loss of strategically placed neurones is accompanied by defect in particular neurotransmitters: basic ganglia cells and dopamine in one case, cortical and hippocampal cells and acetylcholine and choline acetyltransferase in the other. Nor is it clear which comes first, the cell loss or the chemical defect, for the cortical cell loss may conceivably be trophic. The limited success obtained in controlling Parkinsonism certainly opens the possibility of a similar attack on Alzheimerism if the analogy holds. Of the two diseases, we know far less about Alzheimerism, simply because it has been mistaken for an inherent manifestation of old age.

It is possible that, as in the case of Parkinsonism, some forms of Alzheimerism result directly from viral infection, either persistent or acting by way of sensitization of immune mechanisms to brain cell protein (Jancovic et al., 1977; Gajdusek, 1974). Whereas in Huntington's chorea and Parkinsonism the changes are localized in the striatum and the substantia nigra, respectively, in Alzheimerism, the mischief is hippocampal and cortical, and there is accumulating evidence that presynaptic acetylcholinergic fibers are chiefly involved (Davis and Maloney, 1976). The designation "senile" is philosophically unjustified except as a descriptive term, because although a few plaques may be observed in the brains of most very old subjects, Alzheimerism as a definite syndrome is not, nor does choline acetyltransferase decline with normal aging. Huntington's chorea, which is also a genetically determined abiotrophy with a long latent period, would have been regarded as senile if its latency had been substantially longer.

The genetic association of Alzheimerism in relatives of patients with Down's syndrome and with hematologic malignancy is interesting, because subjects with Down's syndrome commonly develop Alzheimer-like changes at an early age and are at high risk from leukemias. Microtubular disorganization has been suggested as a common basis, on the grounds that it, too, is increased by aging processes. Leakage of tubule protein with the eventual appearance of autoimmunity is another possibility, and much work has been done on the association of Alzheimerism with chromosomal abnormalities (Jarvik et al., 1971; Jarvik, 1974). In any analysis of the genetic basis of predisposition, the high incidence in Down's syndrome is something of a conundrum, since the risk to first-degree relatives of Down's syndrome pa tients, half of whom should inherit one defective gene, is low by comparison with expectation.

Choice between possible chain-of-events models is complicated by the virtual impossibility of prospective studies, but from the clinical point of view, the most identifiable and potentially modifiable lesion appears to be a massive decline in choline acetyltransferase (CAT) and acetyl cholinesterase (AChE) in the hippocampus, amygdala, and cortex (Bowen, 1977). It is possible that this change directly reflects loss either of cells or of synapses. On the other hand, judging from the results in palliating Parkinsonism by the supply of deficient dopamine, attempts to supply acetylcholine or to reduce its degradation seem abundantly justified. Choline supplied in the diet had a small but noticeable effect on the dementing process (Boyd et al., 1977; Signoret et al., 1978), but because far higher and more sustained blood levels can be achieved with dietary lecithin (Wurtmann et al., 1977), this would appear to be the test material of first choice (Perry et al., 1977). Missing from the present armamentarium is any serviceable AChE inhibitor not disqualified by its peripheral toxicity which could serve as part of a replacement-conservation or a replacement-neutralization therapy analogous to the combination of levodopa and carbidopa. If centrally selective AChE inhibitors exist, they might be sought among the compounds examined during the development of "irreversible" AChE inhibitors for use as insecticides, or even war gases, but no therapeutic agent of this kind is now available (Comfort, 1978). The low levels of AChE present in the brains of Alzheimer patients are no bar to this approach. They may reflect a reduced number of synaptic sites, but they may equally be a response to low acetylcholine (ACh) levels, a possibility which could be checked if ACh levels could be raised substantially in Alzheimer patients.

A replacement approach would, on the most optimistic estimate, produce palliative results as good as those achieved with levodopa in Parkinsonism, with arrest or partial regression of the dementing process.

The chief ground for therapeutic optimism is that in many cases of chronic brain syndrome, at least in the early stages, the dementing process is primarily an amnesia with which an otherwise fairly intact patient visibly wrestles. There is a considerable resemblance between this process of inaccessibility to recall and the confusional effects of anticholinergic drugs (Drachman, 1974): It may therefore be a matter of neurotransmitter deficit rather than of irrevocable cell loss. The growing recognition of acute symptomatic brain syndrome in older persons, precipitated by infection, medication, and disturbances of electrolyte balance, in which an equally severe or more severe symptomatology is reversible, makes an energetic therapeutic approach to chronic brain syndromes much more credible. How much they can be palliated will not be known until therapeutic experiments are conducted.

Substantial prophylaxis, too, is not an unreasonable hope. An extensive program of neuroendocrine and immunologic studies would be required, preferably longitudinal and concentrated among subjects at apparent genetic risk, since the fundamental changes probably long precede the appearance of dementing symptoms. One way of monitoring early chemical or immune changes which foreshadow eventual Alzheimerism might be to look for them in the only population in which eventual incidence is known, namely, young subjects with Down's syndrome. So long as experiment is limited to harmless materials such as lecithin, there would seem to be no ethical objection to seeing what an attempt to elevate brain ACh levels does to the eventual incidence of Alzheimer-type pathology in Down's syndrome—or, for that matter, to the mental state of Down's syndrome in general, where attention has focused more on tryptophan and serotonin than on ACh metabolism.

Alzheimerism may well turn out to cover a number of pathologies, some of which, like postencephalitic and manganese-induced Parkinsonism, will prove to be epidemiologically identifiable. Among nonviral environmental factors, most geriatric psychiatrists would wish to look at alcohol as a precipitant, but at the moment, direct comparison of drinking with nondrinking communities (Mormon, Pentecostal) is likely to be frustrated by lack of proper postmortem criteria. The brief interest in aluminium toxicity based on the finding of high levels of Al in demented brain (Crapper et al., 1973) appears to have subsided: Al levels are high in senile brain generally and correlate with age rather than with dementia (McDermott et al., 1977). Environmental factors there certainly must be, however, judging from the existence of identical twins discordant for the disease (Hunter et al., 1972). Proper geriatic diagnosis and the demise of the shotgun diagnosis of "senility" to cover all confusional disorders of older people may make epidemiological research easier, but there is more than one dementing process in older people and, at the moment, no substitute for histological examination to differentiate Alzheimerism with certainty.

Although the likelihood is that Alzheimerism is another complex and elusive process like multiple sclerosis, involving immune, genetic, and possibly infective elements in close interplay, there is also the possibility of a far simpler biochemical lesion involving the interaction of vasoactive peptides with the cholinergic system, the model proposed by Bowen (1977). The involvement of vasopressin in cholinergic memory processes seems established (see Legros, 1978; Oliveros, 1978). For the present, it might serve to focus attention on some of the features of Alzheimerism other than the dementia—the cachexia which may accompany it, for example—and possible changes in hypothalamic rather than cortical function. The major attitudinal advance has, however, already taken place, in the recognition of late-life cerebral degeneration as a specific, common, and catastrophic disease, the palliation of which would alter the entire image of aging in the public mind.

In many early or mild cases of dementia, the main experiential deficit is loss of recall rather than loss of intellection. In some cases, this is as isolated a symptom as agnosia in stroke, and the patient's self-awareness is intact. He may "shrug off" nonrecognition of faces or getting lost in familiar places, since amnesia extends to the illness itself and such episodes may be forgotten before they can produce anxiety. In these cases, rehabilitation by constant reminder is an important preservative of personal well-being. It can also help to stave off catastrophe-crisis reactions in intellectual patients who feel their impairment of memory acutely. Not all these cases are progressive: In some, a cautiously administered dose of prostigmin can produce striking temporary clarity, suggesting that the loss is as yet wholly chemical, not structural. A closely similar, isolated memory syndrome can be produced in young subjects by scopolamine (Bowen et al., 1977). The most plausible present chemical model for an amnesic onset of dementia progressing to cell loss is that lysosomal cathepsin A is released in abnormal amounts and inactivates angiotensin, which may act as a modulator in both specific octapeptidergic and cholinergic neurones (Phillips and Felix, 1976; Bennett, Arregui, and Snyder, 1976). Recent work is reviewed by Bowen (1978). Amnesia, even if severe, is not an index of irreversible dementia; it is equally found in a number of toxic, confusional, and other conditions. Nor does its presence predict outcome: Tests based on parietal lobe function may do so, however (Hare, 1978).

INFARCTIVE DEMENTIA

It has been clearly shown that "cerebral atherosclerosis" is not a cause of dementia (Hachinski et al., 1974) insofar as cerebral blood flow is concerned. The cerebral blood flow is independently regulated, and reduction sufficient to impair function would require obstruction of nearly all the major afferent vessels. The dementias associated with atheroma are due to multiple embolization. The normal consequence of artery-derived emboli is an overt cerebrovascular accident (CVA). In this case, the embolus is large enough to obstruct a substantial vessel, and subsequent emboli from the same source affect the same vascular territory. To produce dementia, emboli must be small and widespread. This is a relatively rare event compared with stroke: Embolic dementias account for less than 20% of all dementias in the senium (Blessed et al., 1968). It also raises the strong probability that the dementing process may depend less on an embolus shower than on an embolic process in situ, involving red-cell clumping, platelet abnormalities, and similar microvascular events. The ongoing process has for obvious reasons not been observed microscopically: The end result is multiple cavitation with microaneurysm formation. In hypertensive cases (the majority), microhemorrhage followed by infarction appears to be a major cause. Unexplained intellectual decline unaccompanied by frank stroke should not now be attributed to "hardening of brain arteries," in spite of the popular and medical literature upholding this assumption.

Alzheimer-type dementia is characterized by insidious onset (although illness, bereavement, and so on may appear as spurious landmarks for its start) and steady deterioration. Infarctive dementias tend to occur in episodes, with a downward sawtooth course, each episode being marked by an aggravation of signs and symptoms—weakness, slowness, dysarthria, dysphagia, small-stepped gait, exaggerated reflexes, incontinence of affect, and extensor plantar responses. These may subside until the next episode. Each episode leaves the patient more impaired. Infarctive dementia may follow a heart attack.

The best diagnostic aid is to review the case using Hachinski's scoring method (see Table 4.6). Early diagnosis is important, because of the possibility that intervention may arrest the embolic process before damage is irreversible. Infarctive patients are more commonly aware of, and disturbed by, their impairment of function than Alzheimer patients, and accordingly more liable

TABLE 4.6. Diagnostic Index Score for Embolic Dementia

Item	Score
Abrupt onset	2
History of strokes	2
Fluctuating course	2
Focal CNS symptoms	2
Focal CNS signs	2
Stepwise deterioration	1
Nocturnal confusion	1
Relative preservation of personality	1
Depression	1
Somatic complaints	1
Emotional incontinence	1
History of hypertension	1
Evidence of atherosclerosis	1

The higher the aggregate score, the more likely the diagnosis of infarctive dementia. Scores in excess of 7 are diagnostic.
From Hachinski, V.C. et al. (1974).

to acting out and catastrophe crisis in the early stages. A history of these reactions should lead to energetic therapy.

Multiembolic dementias represent a smaller fraction of senile dementias than the Alzheimer group, but one that should be accessible to prevention if not to arrest. The main reason for their present bad prognosis is the inertia with which clinical researchers have regarded them. There is an urgent need for prospective studies, in relation to hypertension and changes in platelet behavior, and for detailed clinical chemistry in the areas of angiotensin physiology, prostaglandins, and coagulation studies in correctly diagnosed cases. At present, most dementias attributed to "hardening of the arteries" are either secondary (and in some cases curable) or represent Alzheimerism. Another group may be associated not so much with cell loss as with exaggeration of the normal age decline in intercellular synapses (Scheibel and Scheibel, 1975), whether intrinsic or secondary to changes in neurotransmitters. The action of ergot alkaloids, which were originally tried as "cerebral vasodilators," may well depend upon a capacity to alter the metabolism of cAMP or some other important system, but whether the rather irregular benefits they produce in many types of dementia are related to action on neurotransmission, red-cell aggregation, or both has not been established (Yesavage et al., 1979) (See Table 4.7).

Sudden global amnesia in the old is a rare but distinct entity that must be distinguished from fugues and hysterical memory loss in younger patients. The average age of onset is about 64 years, with a range of 49 to 80, the short-term outcome is benign, and most cases have no sequelae, although recurrence, stroke, or dementia are described (Nausieda and Sherman, 1979). The most credible explanation is that it is a transient ischemic attack affecting short-term memory centers, and the best prophylactic treatment against further mischief is that of transient ischemic attacks (TIAs) in general (Olsson et al., 1976). Various studies have given varying incidences of subsequent irreversible damage, but with platelet aggregation inhibitors, the prognosis appears to be good. Sexual intercourse is an occasional precipitant of transient amnesia, sometimes on a single, unexplained occasion (Mayeux, 1979).

Because of the nature of the embolic process and the physiology of brain vessels, vasodilators are predictably ineffective in influencing embolic dementia; although brain—vascular homeostasis does deteriorate with age, this is less a matter of atheromatous insufficiency than a result of fundamental changes in the regulatory ability of angiotensin II (Barker, 1976). Although all anticoagulant therapy is potentially hazardous, this is one form of dementia in which anticoagulants occasionally produce striking improvement (Walsh and Walsh, 1974; Walsh et al., 1978): Some guide to its use can be obtained from the pathology of the dementia. In the early stages, when disease is limited and embolic, the risk could be offset against the prevention of further embolism in situ. At later stages, when cavitation and microhemorrhage have occurred, anticoagulants might be expected to make matters worse. Coumadin appears to be reasonably safe, but it would be rational to evaluate aspirin and sulfin-

TABLE 4.7. Summary of Clinical Studies of Mixed-Effect Drugs and of Primary Vasodilators in Senile Dementias

Drug	Trials		Improvement		No improvement
	Class[a]	Number	Test scale	Practical	
Primary vasodilators					
Cyclandelate	A	7	6	3	1
n = 18	B	2	2		
	C	9	9	6	
Papaverine	A	9	6	1	3
n = 13	C	4	4	2	
Isoxsuprine	A	3	2		1
n = 5	C	2	2	2	
Cinnarizine	A	3	3	2	
n = 8	B	2	2	2	
	C	3	3	3	
Mixed-effect drugs					
Dihydroergotoxin	A	22	22	18	1
n = 33	B	1			
	C	10	10	10	
Nafronyl	A	7	7	7	
n = 8	B	1	1	1	
Pyritinol	A	1	1	1	
n = 5	C	4	4	4	
Pentifylline	A	1	1	1	
n = 12	C	11	11	11	

[a] Class A reports meet all conditions for well-controlled trials; Class B reports are controlled comparisons but are single blind or deficient in one criterion; Class C reports are deficient in two or more criteria or are not controlled.
From Yesavage, J.A. et al. (1979).

pyrazone, on the basis that in situ embolism from red-cell clumping is probably a major factor. The studies by Walsh et al. (1978), although anecdotal in that the full findings in his demented patients were not presented, did include striking improvement in some apparently very deteriorated cases and failure in much milder ones. This work deserves more extensive and systematic confirmation, since the effects of "reality orientation" and enriched activity alone (i.e., a form of psychotherapy, which Walsh's regimen includes) can on occasion be equally striking in the apparently demented.

In the meantime, cyclandelate, which is a "cerebral vasodilator" judged by radioangiography (Eichhorn, 1965), rheoencephalography (Luisada and Jacobs, 1969), and xenon washout (O'Brien and Veall, 1966), has some support as an effective agent to improve mental function and may alleviate some symptoms in dementias of the microembolic type. To have any possibility of clinical success, treatment must be begun early (Birkett, 1971; Judge et al., 1973). Blood flow, however, has been shown to have little relation to symptomatology or its absence in old people (Dekoninck et al., 1977). The beneficial effect of cyclandelate in several types of dementia is almost certainly due to some other action, but appears to be real, and is possibly superior to that of papaverine (Rao et al., 1977). (For a review of other experimental therapies, see Yesavage et al., 1979.) Studies in this area have been plagued by design problems, and the literature, including makers' literature, should be read with caution pending better evidence of benefit.

In distinguishing types of dementia, it is important also to remember that brain damage appears to be additive, so that a normally functioning or minimally demented patient with some brain-cell loss may be pushed into clinical dementia by alcohol damage, a minor stroke, or any other process which causes residual function to be reduced. Misjudged medication, e.g., with antihypertensives, can be such an additional insult.

In susceptible people, alcohol consumption alone can lead to significant brain damage (Brewer and Perrett, 1971). The incidence of chronic brain damage in alcoholics by the mean age of 45 was 5.4% for continuous and 3.3% for intermittent drinkers (Ashley et al., 1976), but the figures increase sharply at higher ages, as brain tissue becomes more vulnerable. In much younger drinkers, the recovery time for psychometric tests with abstinence is at least ten weeks (Clarke and Haughton, 1975); after a long period of addiction, deficits become chronic, although there is evidence that they are reversible by abstinence.

Alcohol is the only common substance of abuse which regularly induces chronic brain damage (Grant and Mohns, 1975). In many longtime drinkers, CNS deficits are more evident than specific intellectual damage (Tarter, 1975). The determinants appear to be individual susceptibility and thiamine deficiency. Fully fledged alcoholic dementia presents with the Wernicke—Korsakoff complex of symptoms (Victor et al., 1971)—ocular palsy, nystagmus, ataxia, amnesia with confabulation, and perceptual and conceptual impairment. But this is only half the story, in that alcohol is the additional insult in a large number of other dementing processes: Although the formulation that it "accelerates brain aging" is probably not strictly accurate, it certainly aggravates almost all cerebral and mental pathologies commonly associated with aging. In infarctive dementia with depression, a single alcoholic episode can induce striking deterioration to the point of virtual decerebration: This appears to be a direct toxic influence of the alcohol itself rather than mediated by thiamine depletion. The interaction of alcohol abuse, "social drinking," and mental illness is complicated, however, by the fact that where depressive symptoms occur as a precursor of dementia, the process becomes circular.

Established alcoholic dementia, like delirium tremens or alcoholic hallucinosis in old subjects, fails as a rule to respond to thiamine though, oddly enough, it has been reported to respond to anticoagulant therapy (Walsh and Lukas, 1974). It can be arrested to some extent, if diagnosed before the full Wernicke—Korsakoff syndrome is present, by withdrawal of alcohol, which is less difficult as a rule in older than in younger subjects, although the risk of delirium and convulsion is always present if intake has been high and continuous. Very often withdrawal exposes an underlying lifelong personality disorder or a depressive state which was the basis of the original alcohol addiction. Liver damage may at this stage make drug therapy hazardous, or ineffective by reason of microsomal enzyme induction. In many respects, therefore, alcohol in twentieth century geropsychiatry occupies the role which was taken by syphilis in nineteenth century alienism. It is the constant complicating factor in all manner of pathologies, and it must always be excluded before diagnosis and treatment are begun for other conditions. This alone is a good enough reason not to regard alcohol as a safe geriatric sedative or a "geriatric wonder drug," in spite of its social acceptance (Stotsky, 1975). Forty-four percent of geropsychiatric patients in one study (Gaitz and Baer, 1971) suffered from concurrent alcoholism. No other drug of addiction is consistently pushed by society and by the patient's friends: There is little excuse for the physician to add to this pressure by pushing it on therapeutic grounds when other more controllable medications are to hand.

The differential diagnosis of organic dementia must always include physical sources of confusion or delirium, medication, undiagnosed depression with withdrawal, and psychotic illness. All but the last of these can affect memory—medication with anticholinergics in particular—but isolated memory deficit with testable performance deficits not due to preoccupation or general confusion is evidence presumptive of organicity. Moreover, all of the conditions which call for exclusion can coexist with organic brain disease: Dementia can occur in people who are eccentric, psychotic, liable to depression, or with major personality difficulties, and their past experience and set will be expressed in the mental changes which organicity brings about. Loss of brain functions will reduce a capacity for social adjustment which is already precarious and will appear not as a personality change but as a rapid aggravation of previous personality difficulties—mania, psychotic decompensation, increased heavy drinking, or sexual indiscretion. Since many of these patients will be admitted as a crisis procedure, organicity can be missed, although it will soon become evident (it would be missed more often but for the mistaken conviction among some admitting officers that all decompensatory behavior in later life is "senile").

Previous personality difficulties are accordingly a poor guide to organicity. When organic change supervenes in a personality problem, the patient's idiosyncrasies are usually exaggerated, and social decompensation indistinguishable from psychosis may result.

A 55-year-old divorced engineer was put on compulsory sick leave by his employer. His work had deteriorated: He would present himself for the wrong shift and work on the wrong machine. The patient had no complaint, except that the foreman was "on his ass" and that he was growing old. Because of this conviction he had consulted a spiritualist. At the age of 50, he had contemplated suicide, but had abandoned the idea because he had read a book dealing with after-death experiences. He had always been a loner, and his wife had divorced him after ten years of marriage because of his dullness and taciturnity. His recreations were model trains and the meticulous writing of extremely neat volumes dealing with psychological topics such as the nature of virility. The matter of these writings showed evidence of much reading: It was preoccupied and odd but not psychotic. Prior to admission, he had been living with a young prostitute, whom he proposed to marry. Self-care had deteriorated, and the house was full of pornographic magazines and bowls of stale cat food. He had attempted to raise $20,000 to buy his mistress a Ferrari sports car.

The patient's appearance was neat, he invariably wore the same outfit. He answered questions in a low voice with much perseveration and appeared to be withdrawn. His only emotion was in reference to the loss of his wife and his hatred for her new husband. On testing, his remote memory was intact but recent memory impaired, and he was mildly disoriented to time but not to person or place. On digit recall, interpretation of proverbs, and simple arithmetic, his performance was grossly impaired: He would shift from addition to subtraction during the course of a problem, but his writing and drawing skills were unaffected. He was not overtly deluded or hallucinated, but gave the impression of deeply preoccupied depression. The only neurological signs were of incipient Parkinsonism, which subsided when antipsychotics were withdrawn.

Within five months of admission, he had moved from taciturnity to complete mutism. CAT scan showed gross general cortical atrophy with numerous "motheaten" translucent areas in both frontal lobes. EEG showed mildly abnormal, scattered 4–7 cps medium-voltage activity during waking state, but no focal abnormality. In spite of the atrophy, no ventricular enlargement could be seen. Four months after admission, his "speech" was reduced to unvoiced lip movement, but he was able to speak and occasionally named the physician correctly. His appearance was of total inner preoccupation—change of posture in his chair, sighing, gait and body movements were normal and spontaneous. He could repeat a name at 10 minutes and identify three objects in five, naming them almost without phonation. He presented the characteristic picture of abulia and "inner absence" of severe frontal lobe deficit, and the provisional clinical diagnosis was of Pick's disease.

In the light of hindsight, this case history does not tell the entire story. There was indeed early evidence of intellectual impairment; nevertheless, the presentation appeared psychotic, and there was much talk at case conferences of decompensation in an anxious obsessional patient, homosexual panic, and other psychodynamic explanations for his increasingly impaired behavior. Trial of antipsychotics and of antidepressants can indeed be justified in such cases, even in the face of definite organicity. Moreover, since the patient has only one mind, the content of his life experience will be expressed just as much in any organic mental illness as in so-called functional psychosis. In either case, idiosyncrasy of experience reflects an idiosyncrasy of brain function rather than the other way around.

The "happy wanderer" can be easier to diagnose, even if memory deficit is not prominent. In some cases, incipient cerebral atrophy can mimic mania, especially if activity and loquacity are unremitting.

> Mr. F. was a still-robust, talkative man of 82, rather reminiscent of Popeye the Sailorman. His main topic of complaint to the psychiatrist was his need for podiatry and the fact that when he ate, his food "sank down" into his calves. He was boisterously anecdotal, with pressure of speech and flight of ideas, and some idioglossia—telling stories, playing to the gallery at consultation rounds, and anxious to demonstrate his physical fitness and ability to stand on his head. He had exhausted many successive relatives. One had the impression of a rich fantasy life based on shifting confabulatory delusions. He was referred because of wandering and well-concealed memory loss.
>
> Mr. F.'s dementia was of a piece with his style: He had indeed run away to sea to avoid a bullying father, and his obsession with "fresh air" was quite in keeping. His preoccupation with physique was of long standing, and his awareness of aging seemed to be making his manic defense against threats to this more urgent. Lithium and antipsychotics did him no good: On further testing, there was gross memory deficit and evidence of extensive cortical atrophy. In long-term care, dementia gradually replaced volubility, but it was patchy, and his interest in life remained.

Although the march of organic dementia cannot as a rule be arrested, its effects can be palliated by sensory stimulation and so-called reality orientation (Brook, 1975). More correctly, perhaps, they can be grossly aggravated, or even induced in old people who are not demented, by withdrawal of activity and sensory input (Ernst et al., 1977), a form of mischief for which the typical custodial institution is ideally suited. This process may be precipitated by the diagnosis of dementia, which leads the staff to give up trying. Sensory stimulation for the old person with brain damage does not mean harrassment to "participate" or a round of frenzied organized activity. The most useful means are continual repetition of ordinary information (the date, people's names, items of current news) and continued treatment as a participant (Folsom, 1968). Orientation can be assisted, for example, by painting different floors of the building in different colors, providing a large clock and calendar in every room, wearing large name badges, and nondiscouragement of habitual activities, even if these are limited and repetitive, combined with organized and regular, predominantly social, group therapy. Sensory deficit such as deafness, which acts on orientation very like experimental sensory deprivation and is actively hallucinogenic, should be corrected. Medication should be minimal and should not include sedatives. Where community volunteers are available, or old mentally infirm patients can be unobtrusively mixed, during occupational activities for example, with younger patients undergoing physical rehabilitation, a family atmosphere can be created. At Baycrest Hospital in Toronto, volunteers were introduced originally to converse with old immigrants who had reverted from English to Russian and Yiddish (a common event in impaired, elderly, foreign language patients) with remarkable benefit to their general alertness and the re-creation of a surrogate family and a surrogate "shtetl" in which regression to childhood patterns of relationship was not disorientating. Success of this kind is more difficult in a mixed ethnic setting, but involvement can still be achieved, sometimes better in a well-run institution than where the old person remains with rejecting relatives. Day attendance centers have proved of great value in maintaining the orientation of old brain-impaired patients living with relatives.

Many pharmacological attempts to improve brain function and memory have been made (see Sathanathan and Gershon, 1975; Lehman and Ban, 1975; Yesavage et al., 1979a,b). Most of these are experimental and have no place yet in general practice. Hydergine, with or without papaverine, helps some patients. Most series have shown improvement to be statistically significant overall (Gaitz et al., 1977). The problem is that there is no way of predicting who will benefit: The drug is not a "cerebral vasodilator" nor is "atherosclerotic dementia" a real entity. Hydergine's mode of action is unknown, but may include cAMP or adrenergic receptors. It occasionally increases agitation, but this is rare. For the confused—disturbed patient who wanders, soils, or behaves disruptively, thioridazine or haloperidol may damp down the activity, but a reorientating environment in the early stages is possibly the best prophylactic. The risk of aggravating confusion by medication should be constantly in mind, even when treating to dissipate a suspected coincident depression, since tricyclics in particular can induce gross confusion by anticholinergic action. In any apparently stationary or deteriorating case, frequent drug holidays are essential for reassessment of mental baseline function.

Organic dementia in old age is at present neither curable nor preventable, although in principle it may well prove to be both. In varying degrees, and from all causes including social and remediable, some dementing symptoms probably affect about 10% of all those over 65. Dementias accordingly represent perhaps the most important single drain on community health resources and certainly the most demoralizing threat to the aging person. The prevention of iatrogenic and nursing-home dementias alone by the provision of proper geriatric services, which has been shown by European example to be perfectly feasible, would reduce the economic cost by a large figure; a radical scientific attack on embolic and Alzheimer-type dementias by a larger figure still. The conclusions to be drawn from these facts are inescapable.

5

TESTS AND TESTING

The mental tests which the physician will encounter in the diagnosis of old-age problems are of several kinds. General tests of function and orientation enable the doctor to check whether the patient has signs or symptoms of confusion, memory loss, and the like. Diagnostic tests are used to discriminate between organic and other causes of dysfunction, to pinpoint and measure specific important disabilities, and to indicate what manner of person the patient is. Beside these, there are various "inventories" (to be filled out by the observer, not the patient) which are used to codify state and progress, such as the Sandoz Geriatric Assessment Scale (SCAG) (Shader et al., 1974) and the nursing observation scale (NOSIE). Some of these can be very useful to plot clinical impressions, and grossly misleading if the results are treated statistically as if they were objective measurements comparable with blood sugar or rainfall levels.

For further diagnosis, and in particular when attempting to discriminate between different psychoses and between psychoses generally and organic dementia, there is a vast range of psychometric tests available which are the province of the clinical psychologist. Performance tests examine specific capacities (the Wechsler Adult Intelligence Scale (WAIS); the Raven progressive matrices, so-called "intelligence" tests, tests of coordination or perceptual deficit). Personality tests help the physician to answer the question, "What kind of person?" through yes–no answers to direct questions about attitudes and experience (the MMPI); through responses to a set of evocative but formless figures (the Rorschach blots), which can be analyzed either statistically or psychoanalytically; through the completion of unfinished phrases, the attachment of a story to equivocal pictures, or free association about threatening or loaded topics. The results may be assessed statistically, or the test material may be used like the Tarot cards to encourage examination of the patient's situation and modes of thought and response. Projective tests are both an indication of what preoccupies the patient and how he treats his preoccupations, and a way of stylizing diagnostic dialogue so that clinical patterns appear and specific concerns or modes of response are uncovered, which can then be pursued in therapy. The invention of new tests (especially of the inventory or scoring variety) is an occupation, like the composition of hymn tunes by organists, which it seems pointless, because impossible, to restrain. The geriatric psychiatrist will find that a few established and well-tried tests (the WAIS, the MMPI, the modified Bender—Gestalt test as a useful minimum) cover most of his needs, backed by special tests to reveal, for example, aphasia, and neurological tests performed in the office, such as the simultaneous face—hand test for organicity. The initial and chief geriatric use of testing is to establish whether there is intellectual dysfunction and whether or not it represents organic brain damage: In addition to strictly psychological tests, the geriatric psychiatrist must also be familiar with the neurological tests for minimal brain dysfunction.

The notion that age is necessarily accompanied by mental blunting dies hard. At the same time, because confusion is a common nonspecific presentation of many geriatric disorders, physical as well as psychiatric, testing is a necessary part of geriatric examination.

Geriatric patients require protection from threatening or impertinent investigation of their mental state. Old people approach tests, to which, compared with the much-tested scholars of today, they are often unaccustomed, with an apprehension born of the folklore of general senility. Before any major tests are instituted, the doctor requires a rough guide to the patient's mental state. At the same time, the first interview can make or mar the therapeutic relationship.

If a standard test such as that of Denham and Jefferys (1972) or Blessed, Tomlinson, and Roth (1968) is used, the already apprehensive older patient may be asked what time it is, what place he is in, and other questions implying imbecility. Much that is harmful about the attitude of the examining physician to older people can be communicated by this procedure. Luckily no such insensitive assault is necessary in the preliminary exclusion of symptomatic confusion from disease or overmedication. Hodkinson (1972) was able to reduce the standard inventory of the Royal College Study to ten questions without loss of discrimination. Many of these coincide with, or approximate, those of a normal admission routine.

With this in mind, the admitting physician can and should expect to obtain an estimate of mental function sufficient (a) to exclude symptomatic confusion and (b) to obtain a guide to disposal and management without risking the hostile reaction which overt mental tests produce in the alert but anxious older patient, if he will divide the material of the Hodkinson inventory between questions normally to be asked of a new patient and questions which test specific capacities, including the first in the history taking and the second in the clinical examination of the CNS. Exclusion of "senile dementia" is not a function of these tests; it will depend on history, exclusion of other causes, and more prolonged observation.

In the first minutes of the interview, the patient is asked name, address, age, year of birth, date of birth, name of next of kin, past or present occupation, and the time of scheduled appointment. Only if the score on these items is less than 7/8 is it necessary to proceed to detailed testing of orientation in time and place, recognition of persons (doctor, nurse) and the like, unless (a) the subsequent course of the history and examination reveal signs of confusion, e.g., between hand and foot, left and right, in response to simple instructions, or (b) there is independent evidence of confusion based on reliable testimony (relatives are reckless in describing the old as "not knowing what they are doing," but specific events such as losing the way should be noted). Where confusion is reported but not complained of, one should ask specifically, "I hear you have had some problems over losing yourself, over getting confused. Is that so?"

Serial performance and 5-minute memory require specific tests. The physician should announce, "I am going to examine your nervous system," and combine these tests with inspection of reflexes and pupils, Wartenburg's head-drop test, and similar unthreatening examinations. The patient is given, among these tests, a phrase or address for 5-minute recall and is asked to count backwards from 20.

The aim of mental impairment tests in geriatrics is the detection of gross disorientation, but even for the detection of finer degrees, and the differentiation of confusion, amnesia, and expressive aphasia, conversation and observation are often superior to tests in forming initial diagnoses and can always be supplemented by them. Although impromptu questions during the history are not statistically standardized, they can be geared to the patient's occupation, educational level, and general style of conversation. It is pointless to test ideation and expression in a truck driver by asking him to distinguish "effect" from "affect," although this in caricature is what some standard tests may do. In the patient's eyes, this reflects on the mental capacity of the physician. By contrast, a question drawn from the patient's experience ("What is the difference between a diesel and a straight motor?") establishes rapport and stimulates response. It has been shown (Gilmore, 1972) that inventory tests and proverb interpretation can give grossly misleading results in old people, exactly as they do in socially underprivileged children, unless they are modified to reflect the patient's past and present experience.

None of the "covert" items contained in history taking is in any way threatening, and time should be taken over them to avoid stressing. Tests of memory and performance specifically grouped with tests of physical function lose much of their threatening character.

Mental loss in age may not be primarily intellectual. Especially in those with paranoid ideation or after a CVA, sensory and cortical loss ranging from deafness to agnosia and aprosopognosia are extremely common, and the symptomatology includes a coping attempt to render life intelligible. Some nominally-aphasic patients can give personal details, but do so in a wooden manner. If this is suspected, object naming must be included in the CNS examination. In this case, the patient asked to name a pencil may say "For writing?"; or a watch, "I used to have one." Rapid recovery of naming on challenge is an excellent index of response to treatment after infarction or toxic confusion from sickness or medication. The "plastic bag test" is mandatory in assessing mental function, where minimal doses of drugs can induce marked transient confusion.

The aim of this approach is not to revise standard psychometric tests used in assessment or psychiatric wards but to reduce the impact of insensitive testing of older patients in the office or the admitting room, and its limitations must be recognized. Simple tests may miss the isolated intellectual symptom (aprosopognosia, for example) or the "armored" early dement who responds mechanically. Such defenses rarely survive a careful history and genuine interpersonal conversation, and rigid tests, by inhibiting the second of these, may actually conceal the diagnosis.

Simple status tests, including a more extensive mental status questionnaire (Wilson and Brass, 1973) can easily be administered by the physician. So can the modified Bender Gestalt test (copying the first three diagrams) and the face—hand simultaneous stimulation test for quick assessment of organicity. More extensive tests should be done by a clinical psychologist, and tests for aphasias by a speech pathologist. The tests require standard administration; they are difficult to interpret, and they present special problems in the elderly, for whom the mere fact of answering all the items in the MMPI questionnaire may represent a considerable task. The doctor who wishes to become skilled in using these and other tests should not only read the literature but also spend time in watching the tests applied. In reassessment, the same tester should review the patient if at all possible. Gedye et al. (1972) developed a teaching-machine type of automated test, using the WAIS in a modified form, and applied it to clinical drug testing. This approach has advantages in removing observer error, and might be extremely useful in serial assessment. But for diagnostic purposes, the standard psychological tests applied by a skilled operator are not replaceable at present. The choice of tests should be decided in consultation with the clinical psychologist: Some units prefer that the psychologist with whom the history has been discussed request particular tests from a colleague, who then performs them blind, but there is little evidence of bias in the normal arrangement.

Mental tests do not supersede clinical impression, but they can sharpen it. They should be considered on a level with all other investigations, and the diagnoses reached should be reviewed constantly in the light of hindsight by the whole ward team, so that the range of results can be matched with particular clinical pictures, otherwise nothing is learned by experience.

Tests must also be selected, from the large number available, for their suitability not only to the old in general but also to the individual patient. The unnecessarily pompous language of the Maudsley Personality Inventory was not intelligible to old, working-class patients (Gilmore, 1972) even with the "translation" thoughtfully provided by its author: One old lady faced with question H ("Are you inclined to be quick and sure in your actions?") replied that it was "too hifalutin a question." Glasgow elderly for whom "rates" mean city taxes and nothing else were confused by question J ("Would you rate yourself a lively individual?"), which is hardly idiomatic English by any standard. In any questionnaire-type inventory, old people are less biddable as a group in giving yes—no answers; they tend to qualify them, often feistily ("I used to, but now I don't get the chance"; "I would, if people would let me"; or even "I can't trust anyone nowadays."). Tests which are perceived as childish, such as Raven block tests, may give rise to strong reactions or uncooperative disinterest. Experience with a given population will show which of these are better dropped in favor of others seen as not demeaning.

6

GERIATRIC PSYCHOTHERAPY

AGING AND THE PHYSICIAN

Some understanding of the inner experience of aging is necessary to all physicians, even if their time to practice direct psychotherapy is limited. They need to understand the patient's feelings, if only to communicate effectively, and to direct the brief psychotherapy implicit in every doctor—patient interview. We all have difficulty in appreciating what old age will be like, but the physician may have peculiar difficulties in addressing it which arise from countertransference, the covert feelings aroused in the practitioner by the patient.

It helps in both undertakings if we recognize that one of the most fundamental questions in the psychiatric dialectic is: "What are this person's sources of self-value?" Human life involves a number of potential sources of self-esteem, and threats to it which present as anxiety. Some are unconscious and derived from childhood; others, conscious, derived from our experience of living, and often realistic. One of the most important of "existential" anxieties is the knowledge that human life is limited by death. In dealing with such sources of unease, there are sources of consolation, rational and irrational, which are ego-syntonic. Some of these when pursued prove illusory; others, however irrational our intention in following them, prove worthwhile for their own sake. Sources of self-value accordingly range from reaction formations to consciously formulated values, but the boundary between them is always blurred.

Physicians, by reason of the experience of medical training, have to deal with an unvarnished picture of life, including death and suffering, at a relatively immature age, with little opportunity to examine their feelings, and under academic pressure. It is a natural reaction formation to invest much self-esteem in their ability to heal (which is, after all, what the exercise they are engaged in is about). For this reason, patients who are unable to be cured, by threatening our adjustment, are doubly castrating: They manage at one and the same time to resist our ability to heal and to remind us of our own eventual death. This destabilizing effect is seen in the terminally ill, whom we may avoid or treat by officious overmedication and denial, and in the old, who are a threatening prospectus for our own later years.

With the introduction into medical schools of planned sessions in which students are given skilled help in facing these difficult experiences and emotions early on, they can be made manageable by being brought into the open. Of those who had no such opportunity, some may react by overt hostility to the old. Most of us have had experience of the occasional teacher whose reaction formation was hard-nosed realism and who stressed the uselessness and the nonresponse to treatment of persons over 50, 60, or 70 (the cut-off age becomes noticeably higher as the speaker ages). Contact with good geriatric medicine will rapidly dissipate such notions about the untreatability of the old, but the soft-nosed geriatrician whose security rests in an unconscious denial that physical aging, dementia, and, by implication, death have any reality, since they can always be "cured," is in no better shape, for he may react with equal hostility or avoidance toward the patient who calls the denial into question by the obvious reality of his decline.

> A retired physician who lived in a residential home was very concerned about the behavior of the young, recently appointed, physician in charge. Always inclined to be brusque and patronizing toward the patients, this man had the habit of muttering to himself while making his rounds, "Jesus, how I hate old people!" His motives in volunteering for a post which involved looking after old people as a fulltime activity had not been explored. His elderly colleague was more concerned about this unprofessional conduct than about the risk that the young man might prove to be psychotic.
>
> The matter was raised with the proprietors: Their reaction was that the young doctor was well recommended and professionally competent and kept a tight ship, and they saw no reason to intervene.

Introspection by the physician of his own countertransference toward any patients he finds difficult or disquieting is a personal matter, but salutary. If not conducted during undergraduate clinical study, it can profitably be undertaken at any age with the help of a psychiatric colleague. Meanwhile, any physician who has charge of a geriatric ward will inevitably be engaged in considerable psychotherapy with nursing and junior staff: their disturbance at the actual or impending death of a patient; their feelings of anger toward angry and unresponsive patients, who have their own problems and decline to respond to tender loving care, and toward the relative slowness of age. Self-confrontation is necessary in order to handle these difficulties in others. It is also sometimes necessary to point out that the hospital is there to make the patients, not the staff, feel better.

AGE AND THE PATIENT

The difficulties which we ourselves encounter in addressing age professionally are a good psychiatric preamble to the problems of the old. Age is inevitably, even in the most fortunate, a period of loss. It has compensations, but in an anti-old society, these are few compared with the resources of some simpler orders, and in any case, one only asks for compensation if one has been run over. Age can, with luck and a robust personality, be a time of enjoyment; at the same time, nobody would wish to be physically old if they had the choice of being young.

The sources of self-value in different individuals differ greatly in nature and in realism. Sexual desirability, strength, work performance, ability to get and retain possessions, production of children, artistic skill and reputation, independence, and even relatively trifling skills such as the ability to win at golf may be significant to different people. Most or all of these may be compromised by age changes. Some such as child bearing inevitably are; others persist. Creative activities, which are basically inner directed but win applause ("Fame, wealth and the love of women" in Freud's formulation of the aims of the artist), stand up best, failing complete decrepitude. Demonically creative people, the Picassos and Furchtwanglers of this world, age well and see sickness and death chiefly as annoying interruptions of their creativity. Not all of us are so lucky. Investment in friends, kin, and spouses is threatened by bereavement, in progeny by the menopause, in sexual desirability by decline in physical beauty or "manliness," in work by retirement, and in skills or performance by weakness or by neurological deficit.

At the same time, age is rarely experienced primarily as change in the self: The transformation is in others, and in the manner in which the old person is treated. These changes may produce something akin to bewilderment, a sensation of being bewitched. The experience is that of Rip van Winkle— others have aged, and young others now treat us as old.

These feelings are rarely expressed directly by older people, but they are commonly expressed indirectly, often by the content of dreams or of symptoms. In most people, adjustment is made to the changed mode of living, but the possibility of making it with success depends on the robustness of self-valuation and its independence of vulnerable attributes such as physical beauty or professional status. The greater the investment in such props to self-esteem, the less they can be retrospective: What has been achieved has little capacity to support the present sense of worth, and the fact of no longer achieving can actually damage it.

The ability to come to terms with altered capacities without loss of self-esteem and without rekindling anxieties depends also upon luck. All too often, the older person succumbs to a general assault by misfortune—his or her own or a spouse's disabling illness, with dependency, role loss, financial hardship, and an awareness of being unwanted or burdensome. This commonly follows, for example, a CVA. It may also commonly occur at the moment when the patient has retired and is attempting to substitute a new source of satisfaction "in doing things he or she had always wanted to do." In these circumstances, the reaction is anger. The catastrophe is experienced as undeserved punishment. Whereas younger patients threatened by death quite often "bargain with God" for recovery, the old patient beset by multiple interrelated disasters exhibits a Job-like indignation with Providence for which there is no approved outlet in the culture: We do not encourage the unfortunate to be angry. Some patients deal with anger by denial and religiose resignation, and others by depression or irritability, but even minimal and transient brain impairment may allow the full intensity of the patient's indignation to be expressed, often at relatives and staff, who are threatened and upset by it. Recognition of this may play a useful part in family counseling and staff discussion. Permission to experience or express anger is a key procedure in the reconstructive psychotherapy of many old and all terminal patients, during which the therapist may expect to serve as scapegoat, not only, as in conventional analytically based therapy, for parent figures, but also for children and for Providence.

We have found some of these considerations more valuable in the interpretation of distress among older patients than the analysis of childhood experiences by which the anxieties and the choice of reaction formation were determined. By the geriatric age, sources of self-value have become functionally autonomous: There is little mileage to be got out of changing them, but with supportive therapy, they can be supplemented. In fact, by giving permission, the psychiatrist can sometimes enable unreasonable self-demand to be relaxed, using age as a pretext, with a striking increase in contentment and well-being.

The expectation of dysphoria with age and society's tolerance of somatization as opposed to its intolerance of unhappiness are particularly important in later life. One may not say that life is a pain in the neck, but one may have a pain in the neck. Society reinforces the secondary gains of somatization. Other socially determined and normally unexpressed attitudes which come home to roost in age are the American philosophy of independence and achievement coupled with high mobility, the valuation of society as a competitive bear garden in which the unfortunate or unsuccessful are so through their own fault (the obverse, it would appear, of the positive valuation of effort and equal opportunity), the assiduously cultivated view that community support is enervating and its acceptance demeaning, and the popular mythology of sexual performance as a personal validation and its decline as a feature of age. We have overfocused on the psychosocial problems of the young as indices of stress and irrationality in society. The psychosocial problems of the old are probably a much better index of the humanly inviable points in a national ideology: Old people are those who have lived by that ideology, while the young are still trying to deform themselves to fit it. Geriatric psychiatry is accordingly an instructive discipline for those who practice it, and would be so for social ideologues were they educable by experience.

The attitude of society to age and the involvement of aging with losses of many kinds virtually guarantee that all geriatric treatment is "psychotherapy." Formal psychotherapy of deliberate intent most commonly opens with crisis intervention, often in response to bereavement, desertion, or illness, and its initial aim is support. This does not mean that lifelong problems with self and with others cannot be addressed, and very often resolved. Resolution, moreover, does not necessarily involve a deeply historical attack on early childhood. By the time patients have lived this long, there is a strong tendency for resentments and failures to be conscious and there will be a long record of, for example, self-destructive behaviors, from which the patient can easily be led to recognize his or her own past form. The main difference between treating young and old is probably that with the old, the therapist's commitment is indefinite. They can always be helped, sometimes "cured," and they can be transferred, provided an anchor person acceptable to the patient is provided, but they cannot as a rule be simply discharged. Support mechanisms for the old are so limited in our culture that someone must be available upon whom they can call, either through monthly visits or, quite often, by telephone. In contrast, initial results tend to be rather more rapidly obtained than in young people because problems are clear cut and evident, the life record is available to doctor and patient ("reminiscence therapy" is a powerful resource), and there is no initial beating about the bush to find out what it is that the patient needs, wants, or expects. Often he or she expects very little and starts with a healthy distrust of psychiatrists as persons likely to assume that "the old" are crazy, and with whom consultation is itself a risky admission. Once reassured on this count, they benefit from their surprise and pleasure at finding that the physician respects them.

The traditional and intuitive social reintegrator for the problems of loss in age is respect. This is something which cannot be fabricated and which our society totally discounts. More realistic and more in line with our own mores is the assertion of equality, and this is probably what the geriatric psychiatrist should project. Nobody should need to apologize for being old any more than he or she need apologize for being black or an immigrant. The sense of continuing identity and personal constancy, which is what normal people experience inwardly with aging but find denied by society, can only be reinforced by a physician to whom that sense comes naturally. The psychiatrist who is old may do this effortlessly, because doctor and patient share the experience of time, and the counselor's continuing professional activity is itself a reinforcement to others who feel their function threatened by idleness or denigration. When younger people learn effective geriatrics, they must combine equality with respect and liking in order to avoid being identified by their patients with a world which, on an unconscious if not a conscious level, the old experience as rejecting. Robust older people have skills of self-defense and will answer back when confronted with a Hippocratic oaf, but it is precisely the weak or the uncertain who come for psychiatric help, and immense mischief may be done here by brashness or childrenization. Given a concerned and stable personality in the therapist, however, youth is no bar, and the identification with children or grandchildren may be as therapeutically useful as the identification by younger patients of the doctor as a parent figure. The seeking now is less, or not only, for permission and approval. It is chiefly for validation and love, and this can be projected in an entirely unsentimental way.

Sensitivity to the "self-value" model can also suggest specific therapeutic measures. The craftsman with a physical defect who "cannot stand the sight of his tools," although he still keeps them in order, is a candidate for full occupational rehabilitation even though he is retired. Those who can no longer themselves do can derive self-esteem from acting as instructors, a traditional role for the old in almost all cultures except our own. Often it is better to look for new sources of self-value to replace old—grandparenthood in place of parenthood, for example. In no case should older persons be deprived of demand and function, as they are in many nursing homes. The risk of scalding should not outweigh the therapeutic value of being allowed to make tea for other patients, and the policy of "better not" should be firmly discouraged. As much as half the psychotherapist's work may need to be devoted to the attitudes of staff or family in order to keep the environment in step with the needs of the patient and to prevent acting out at his or her expense.

Fortitude is a neglected psychiatric phenomenon. We recognize it in patients, and tend to like patients who display it, but it remains difficult to answer, other than with platitudes, any question as to why some people, like Beethoven, "take life by the throat" and remain stable in horrendous circumstances while others are destroyed by minimal adversity. It is an immense asset to those who genuinely possess it. It should not be confused with denial or overcompensatory optimism. One would wish to help patients achieve fortitude, and to possess it ourselves, particularly in old age. The cultural prescription of uncomplaining stoicism (the "stiff upper lip") has been actively unhelpful, and one cannot inculcate true fortitude by prescribing it, or disliking patients who lack it. At the same time, it is increasingly necessary to restrain staff members and colleagues who regard the violent expression of emotion as an inherent good and who measure therapeutic progress rather as some Victorian preachers measured the sincerity of conversion, by the loudness and frequency of abreaction. There are indeed those who suppress emotion to their hurt, but there are also those whose self-esteem depends on being in control and who remain so out of self-respect rather than out of fear of losing that control. The old and the young may indeed need to be helped to express grief, anger, hostility, and disappointment, but particularly in the old, these expressions need not be spectacular, no tears may be shed. We should neither react critically to those whose control genuinely fails nor—and this is now a more common error among junior counselors—be disappointed if we cannot induce an emotional response beyond the calm statement of feelings. As one old lady said, "She keeps telling me I don't cry enough. I don't think so."

NEUROSIS AND AGE

A patient who was neurotic when young will be neurotic when old. The style of our response does not change with age, although its degree may become more frantic as options are withdrawn. In previous periods, the climacterics at which irrational or inappropriate modes of dealing with decision-making were exposed tended to be adolescence and young adulthood, in connection with mate selection and employment. Longer life has added a second identity crisis in late middle age. This crisis coincides with the menopause in women, when fertility ends. There is no comparable rite de passage in men, but the experience is similar. In adolescence we find out "who we are" by setting goals which include the preservation of positive childhood experiences (praise from parents, for example) and the realization of experiences which have so far been denied us. In late-life crisis, we have to face "who we have been" and the fact that some fantasies have collapsed on us through nonrealization and others have proved disappointing when realized.

Midlife crisis precedes the geriatric age, but in geriatric psychotherapy, we are dealing with its sequelae. Fantasy goals are now limited by the reduction in the sense of futurity (we are running out of runway), real limitations and bad choices have to be faced, but worst of all, the positive gains—skills, relationships, status, valuation by others, and the prospect of setting right what has gone amiss—all begin to be threatened. Patients whose responses were always exaggerated or inappropriate may be confronted with the results of unwise "now or never" behavior in middle age; stable and wise patients may find that the structure of stability they have built up and relied upon is becoming unstable or collapsing when they lack the strength and resources to repair it.

On this basis one might expect "neurotic" behavior to be increasingly common with age, but this does not seem to be the case (Bergmann, 1978). People who were neurotic before remain neurotic, often with exacerbated symptoms, anxiety disorder being the most persistent (Ernst 1959); what increases with age is, as one might expect, chronicity. But as Bergmann suggests, a prime factor in the transition from being an unhappy person to becoming a sick patient is failure to fulfill role expectations. Age is the time when we are likely to realize that this has occurred; and there is then no time to remedy it. Moreover, because the old in our society have no socially approved role, there is no new agenda which can be substituted for the old one. This situation is enough to make anyone ill. At earlier ages, we may compensate by projecting fantasies into the future. Age is the first time of life when postponement is no longer a cover for failure. It is also the time when death ceases to be a postponable prospect. Not that old people generally are obsessed with the fear of death (this is more often a preoccupation in childhood, adolescence, or young adulthood), but death anxieties play a larger part than psychiatry has usually admitted in the determination of defensive and self-assertive behaviors, and its appearance on the horizon may profoundly affect those behaviors.

In non-neurotic people, fantasy has been transmuted into achievement; they know where they are and who they are. But the sudden confluence of social oldness, loss of work satisfaction, declining stamina, frank illness, and mundane details like poverty, insecurity, and demeaning treatment (which tend to be overlooked in depth-psychological writings about age, but are real enough when one is hit by them) generate not acting out but a sense of stunned or panicky disbelief. The only countervailing factor is that our social image of age is so negative that many old people are agreeably surprised on reaching it to find that they are not demented, sick, incapable of learning, asexual, unemployable, and lonely. Such people may need encouragement in assertion and militancy when they encounter injustice, but they do not become psychiatric patients. It is to the old person, often not previously neurotic, to whom one misfortune happens, that everything tends to happen.

Patients who want counseling are therefore of three kinds: The adjusted old who need help in dealing with the realistic problems which later life brings; the lifelong anxious or unhappy who now react with panic; and those who were doing nicely until, as a result of some unforeseen event, bereavement, illness, or financial miscalculation, everything has collapsed simultaneously. The first benefit from "befriending"; the doctor or the therapy group can act as surrogate kin. The second are patients who need support and specific therapy, either supportive or insight-giving, or both. The third require both of these approaches plus an opportunity to express anger, hurt, and astonishment. Accessory damage from the results of stress—alcoholism in particular—must be dealt with. In all these patients, however, psychotherapy by discussion and personal interchange is neither useless nor unrewarding. Indeed, age may be the first time that these patients have had the opportunity for self-examination with skilled help, or the first time that events have compelled them to seek it.

FAMILY THERAPY

The isolated old person comes to the physician in need of support and in search, effectively, of surrogate kin. Where kin exist, the task can be far more arduous and far less straightforward. The support of the old person has in this case to be offset against the need to deal simultaneously with the emotional difficulties of other family members.

All human family relations are marked by ambivalence, and the age and illness of a parent invariably calls up feelings of hostility as well as concern, and guilt as well as affection. For most people, the gains of the family situation offset the losses, and the geriatrician is justified in looking to the family as an important organ of support, one to which old people have traditionally looked and the lack of which they have traditionally and rightly feared. The mobility and instability of the modern family has reduced this gain and probably exacerbated some of the negatives, but it is still available in many cases.

When the old person presents (or is presented) with frank neurosis, however, caution is in order. Neurotics are not isolated phenomena; they usually have "neurotic" families, in that prolonged interplay with their own personality problems has often evoked reaction in others and a contest of symptomatology has developed. This is particularly so when the patient has parented and reared the adults he or she lives with. The parties will have been honed to a fine degree of fit and have developed an expertise, usually of a negative kind, in exacerbating one another. In this setting, simple relief of the normal ambivalences toward the old, the demanding, and the sick by permission giving and by reinforcement of caring and affection may not be enough.

The patient's behavior—querulous, domineering, manipulative or self-destructive—can often give a clue to what will be found before the relatives are addressed. They may be addressed and found supportive and sensible, but the physician who practices geriatric psychiatry, conducts psychotherapy with a neurotically behaving old person, and then prepares to "see the relatives" may be opening not a dialogue but a can of worms. Old parents who have undergone a reversal of roles by becoming dependent attract all the Freudian unbiddables: guilt, denial or expression of hostility, "undoing" of death wishes by overprotectiveness, together with a variety of end games between complementary personal problems. Extremely menacing material is contained in this situation. It has to be dealt with, since even the temporary removal of the old person to some other setting is a significant intervention and will destabilize other family members, but it rather obviously calls for great caution and is not a suitable training assignment for inexperienced therapy students. Proper management calls for a percipient analysis by the therapist combined with extreme self-control in offering interpretation. Generally the relatives need to be given support in abreacting feelings toward the old person without much comment, but whoever does the counseling will usually end by supporting two or three people without yielding to the temptation to extend the analysis to their general problems (it is the old person who is "the patient")—a situation which in other contexts, such as marital or parent-child counseling, one usually tries to avoid. At some stage, as in couple counseling, all the parties may have to be got together, either on a group-therapy model or with a co-therapist as "advocate" for the kin as the primary therapist is advocate for the patient. This may not always be feasible for practical reasons. If the geriatric psychiatrist conducts family confrontations alone, a *Rashomon* model is in order (after the Japanese film in which each of five parties to a traumatic incident presents his or her own, wholly contradictory version).

Most families are indeed quite capable of ventilating their feelings about and to an older member by guided discussion. The point of the cautions given is that the intensity of these feelings, the ramifications arising from long past history, and the recrudescence in an overt form of childhood difficulties can be unpredictable. Psychiatric literature, which is full of accounts of conflict in childhood, is surprisingly insouciant about the end stages of the relationship, in which a failing parent faces grown-up children. One could learn more from *King Lear* than from most psychiatric textbooks, and proper counseling expertise, both in foreseeing and in dealing with trouble, has still to be documented. Generally speaking, old people with emotional problems may on occasion be far easier to treat if they have no relatives, and some who have do better if they can be detached from them, and their drift into regressive, manipulative, and dependent behaviors reversed. Like all geriatric success, this operation depends wholly on proper social services, psychiatrically expert social workers on whom the doctor can rely, proper housing appropriate to the older person, and sufficient money to meet their needs. Institutions are not the answer, though they can separate the combattants temporarily to their mutual good. Many a family situation inaccessible to counseling has been prized open and made accessible by the physical illness of one of the parties. Such opportunities should be developed for the benefit of all those involved. The psychiatrist who deals with neurotic children is tempted to wish for the abolition of parents; the psychiatrist who has to deal with the neurotic parent grown old might often wish for the abolition of children. Neither is practicable, nor would either improve the situation, but the neurotic old with a neurotic family situation of long standing and the healthy old with severely neurotic kin or associates may benefit as much by a separation as do some children of disturbed parents. In view of the normality of some tension and ambivalence between generations, it requires skill and empathy to determine when family therapy should be directed to overcoming normal frictions and when a radical solution will be needed. This assessment, very like the private assessment made by most marriage counselors when a particular marriage is more destructive than supportive and should not be propped into a sitting posture, can sometimes be made early and therapy directed to enable the parties to dispense with one another. Dissimulation is likely to be greater among the relatives of an old person than between spouses (who are more likely to exaggerate their incompatibilities at the expense of positive elements they take for granted). Vocal tension in the family is a more favorable prognostic sign than exaggerated tolerance and concern. On the other hand, where the family can be enlisted, all parties usually benefit. Accuracy in assessing these complications is a very important skill, not only in frank geriatric psychiatry, whether practiced by physicians or by social workers, but in geriatric as in pediatric medicine.

All interpersonal situations in our culture tend to be affected by the general phenomenon of overexposure—of children to parents, spouse to spouse, and old parents to children or companions—which comes from the model of privacy on which modern living is conducted. There is no equivalent of village society, problems are kept behind doors, and there is no sharing of experience or exposure to criticism and to other than private role models. One of the values of group therapy in reducing problems to size and in offering new strategies is precisely the creation of a nonprivate forum for the ventilation of the home. Both old and young people benefit from this. It also offers an escape route for the therapist where his attempts to help one family member (in this case, the senior member) expose problems in other members, which require assistance but on which he cannot focus in individual therapy. Chapters of "grandparents anonymous" and "relatives anonymous" are apt to arise informally around any geriatric clinic to lighten some of the burdens which privacy adds to an already difficult aspect of relationship. Everything can be addressed here, from unspoken hostility and guilt to differences in standards between generations. How far the severely disturbed senior or relative can benefit will depend on the capacity to take in new attitudes and apply them, but the opportunity should not be denied them.

7

OTHER
PRACTICAL MATTERS

Sleep in the old is an important topic, because of the frequent problems over medication. The psychiatrist may encounter these in discovering iatrogenic confusion from drugs or may be asked to deal with insomnia which disturbs and preoccupies the patient, or institution staff, or both.

In old age, sleep tends to be fragmented rather than continuous, stage 3 and 4 sleep is reduced, without gross changes in REM periods, and individual idiosyncracy of sleep patterns is accentuated. At the same time, old people may spend more time actually sleeping than do the young. For many patients over 70, daytime naps are physiologic, and they should not be disturbed in the interest of night-time sleep.

Insomnia may reflect many processes. Anxiety over sleeping is one of the most common, and growing intolerance to caffeine another, but it can also be found on enquiry to represent dyspnea, anxiety over incontinence, urinary frequency, nocturnal bone and joint pain, and muscle fibrillary spasm. The wakefulness of anxiety (difficulty in getting to sleep) and of depression (early waking, or, occasionally, unrousability and confusion in the morning) require to be distinguished. Chronic anxiety over sleep patterns very often takes origin in a period of crisis which induced wakefulness (bereavement is a very common cause, especially when a relict spouse must now sleep alone); it is then maintained by prolonged use of hypnotics. Institutional nocturnal confusion on admission to hospital, in which a previously unconfused old person wanders in search of the bathroom and does not recognize the change of scene, is often put down to senility, in spite of the fact that it is nearly equally common in small children. The treatment is to wake the patient fully and guide him back to bed. Where this cannot be done, it will usually be found that confusion has been made worse by medication, often a ritual "sleeping pill" given at full young-adult dosage. Phenothiazines occasionally precipitate both nocturnal confusion and sleepwalking (Charnay, 1979). Barbiturates are still demanded by some patients who are used to them and are still prescribed. More than half the prescriptions for barbiturate hypnotics in a recent study were written for persons over 60, who account for 15% of the population (Solomon et al., 1979). Flurazepam, which is perhaps the most used and certainly the most advertised hypnotic benzodiazepin, differs from, for example, oxazepam in that its long-lived active metabolites cumulate with repeated nightly or alternate-nightly dosage, leading to significant impairment both of mental test performance and of skills such as driving (Solomon et al., 1979).

The actual usefulness of *hypnotics* in any age group is in fact very limited. Where the cause of real sleeplessness, as opposed to anxiety about the amount of sleep, is unclear, they may hasten induction and yield an average of 20–40 minutes of additional sleeping time. Where insomnia is due to pain, or where the real problem is depression or dypsnea, better results can be obtained by specific treatment of the causal condition. In rare cases (e.g., sleep apnea), medication of the insomnia is actively life threatening.

All common hypnotics alter the nature of sleep. Although they reduce the latency of stage 1 sleep, most eliminate or reduce REM sleep, stage 3 and 4 sleep, or all of these. With habituation, the shortening of induction and the reduction of waking disappear, after 2–3 weeks of administration, but some degree of REM suppression persists. On withdrawal there is an REM rebound, often with nightmares, and usually with a marked aggravation of fatigue and insomnia. (Chloral hydrate and flurazepam are exceptions, in that they are less apt to produce rebound, and their effect on induction lasts rather longer than with other agents.)

The *treatment of insomnia* consists in proper evaluation, treatment of symptoms which wake the patient, recognition of anxiety and depression, reassurance to the career sleepless who actually sleep adequately, and adjustment of habits (avoidance of coffee, evening excitement, and late meals; non-insistence on scheduled "lights out" when the patient is not ready to sleep; and sometimes suitably timed exercise, massage, or relaxation training). Institutions manufacture insomnia in the old: They are noisy, rigidly scheduled regardless of the large variance in late-life sleep patterns, anxiety producing to the newly admitted, and productive of boredom and lack of fatiguing exercise in the long run. Young patients have the same experiences, but they attract less attention and cause less anxiety and confusion. In general, the greater the enrichment of the environment in later life, the lower the consumption of hypnotics. Withdrawal of orgasm, itself a physiological hypnotic, by absence of a spouse or unwillingness to masturbate in an institutional setting, is quite a common unrecognized factor in insomnia. Anyone who is transferred from a familiar setting to one in which lights may be left on, and in which other persons move about, snore, shout or moan, or even can be felt to be unaccustomedly present, will sleep badly.

Hypnotics are used in the treatment of crisis insomnia, including admission to hospital. Their period of administration should in no case be longer than 14 days, preferably much less, since after that time they do nothing to improve sleep and their effects, especially on the old, are wholly negative. Very low doses of chloral hydrate, flurazepam, or (rarely) butobarbital are appropriate. All these should then be tapered and withdrawn by about the 10th day. They should be supplemented by general measures, including allowing the patient to become normally fatigued by activity, if the illness leading to hospital admission permits, a light night meal, and a hot milk-containing drink. If the patient wakes "hung over," the dose should be reduced, or the drug withdrawn. In spite of ward routine, the habitual home sleep pattern should be (a) ascertained and entered on the notes and (b) preserved, if necessary by allowing the patient to read or listen to radio until ready to sleep, and the nightcap and medication given on demand not at a fixed time; and by not waking the patient at an unaccustomed hour to take breakfast or to have vital signs checked unless this is necessary. If they can do so without disturbing the ward, ambulatory patients should be allowed to get up if wakeful and have a snack.

The insomnia of depression is treated with sedative antidepressants at night. The insomnia of painful terminal illness often responds to a combination of amitryptilene and a sedative antihistamine. Early recourse to opiates may increase tolerance and make them ineffective when really needed. Much can be learned about an institution by examining the Kardex for prescriptions of hypnotics p.r.n., or worse o.n., a finding which indicates the need for radical education of the responsible staff.

In the treatment of night-time confusion in hospital, the most useful "medications" are the installation of a night-light, dim enough to allow sleep but bright enough to show the outlines of the room, careful enquiry into the patient's usual bedtime, and the waiving of all rigid lights out rules; administration of a hot milk drink on demand, followed for a few nights by minimal sedation with chloral or flurazepam if sleep is delayed over 1 hour; and provision of an accessible, convenient commode. In the same way, the best remedies for daytime confusion are regular human contact; the provision of a large, quiet clock and a regularly updated calendar; and regular daily variation of menu, since in an institution, meals are perhaps the most memorable daily events.

Geriatric patients commonly arrive at the hospital armed with supplies of chronically administered hypnotics. Withdrawal of these may be a problem; where doses have been large and administration has lasted over years, a sudden cutoff may precipitate convulsions and will certainly cause anxiety and insomnia. These drugs are commonly multiple and may include highly toxic and confusing prescriptions (glutethimide, methaqualone) which are contraindicated in geriatrics. The first step is to "cannibalize" all sedatives (including alcohol), regardless of chemical constitution, to a single manageable agent and then withdraw that, under cover of small amounts of diazepam or a sedative antihistamine if necessary, with strong psychotherapeutic and explanatory support. The surrender of a beloved pill may of itself cause anxiety, but this is often offset by the striking improvement in memory and well-being which follows reduced medication.

"Goldwyn's syndrome" is the name which has sometimes been flippantly given to disturbance in glorious technicolor, including noisy insomnia. Old people are not "childish," but, like children, they are human. Under stress and deprivation, or when mentally or physically ill, they may resort to attention-seeking behavior. In doing so, they will lay hold of the role we present them and read the cues which produce the most attention. Because "senility" is an available role, some people will exploit its theatrical potential to offset loneliness and impersonal handling by staff. To the child's resources (breath holding, overbreathing, tantrums) and the adult's emotion-signaling repertoire (shouting, swearing, weeping) they may add a special repertoire of dramatized "senile" behavior, including incontinence, and "demented" activities of various kinds, especially those which most upset and threaten the staff.

Floridly disruptive antics may reflect real brain damage, psychosis or mania, or be the endpoint of a lifetime of manipulative behavior (one can imagine Madame Bovary in a nursing home). The trouble is that since with solicitous or even irate staff, attention-seeking behavior is strongly reinforced, a tug-of-war develops. The patient's degree of derangement and disruptive potential is graphically described to the psychiatrist (sometimes in front of the patient). The only way to deal with such understandable but distressing reactions is to give human attention to the full, but without reinforcing the demonstration. Staff are told to withdraw as soon as the curtain rises on the drama and stay away until it falls. As soon as quiet is restored, the patient (who has often been isolated to reduce the audience) should be visited, talked to, touched, and generally dealt with as a human being in good standing. Such attention-giving visits should then be repeated at regular frequent intervals and interrupted only if another performance is scheduled. The physician should expect one or two highly dramatized farewell appearances, often heralded by telephone calls from the ward that "Mr. Jones is playing up again." This usually means that the reinforcement schedule broke down at a particularly loud noise. Staff education should continue until the unwanted behavior is extinguished. The patient, whether mentally ill or not, must then be provided with normal human services of contact and attention without the trouble of adopting extreme measures. Sedation short of unconsciousness is wholly ineffective in such cases; it simply impairs judgment and increases confusion. "The old" are only more prone to attention-seeking behavior than "the young" because of the withdrawal of validation which we impose on them and the wounding dependency which springs from illness or institutionalization. In a milieu in which it is assumed, however tacitly, that they are senile, unapproachable, infantile or "bonkers," the old have few alternatives but to exploit the situation and turn their torments into horrid arms. Some will be more prone to do this than others, but they are not by any means those with whom psychotherapy is the least rewarding.

Hypochrondriasis is more common in late than in early life, since somatic anxieties understandably increase. It, too, is a reinforced behavior, but harder to deal with because the reinforcer is that somatic expressions of anxiety, frustration, and anger are socially acceptable while the emotions are not: Everything conspires to reinforce the secondary gains of illness.

The hypochondriac is an office problem, the patient physicians dread. Failure to respond to authority or to reinforce the doctor by being healed complicate the countertransference. The important psychiatric points are that referral is treated as rejection, the threat of cure is a threat to secondary gains, and the physician is either blamed for failing to effect a cure or made responsible for present illness which the patient attributes to past investigation.

Hypochondriasis as a way of life must be distinguished from somatic anxiety as a feature of depression, because while freestanding hypochondriacs receive support and minimize conflict by ill health and are not suicidal, somatically anxious depressed patients very often kill themselves. The hypochondriac, like Milton's Satan, has a sense of injured merit—responsibility for his sufferings is projected onto others, others are not appropriately sympathetic, only incompetence prevents a cure. His medical knowledge may be volubly expressed. Unlike the patient with Briquet's syndrome, who has florid signs and symptoms but views them with "fine indifference", and the obsessional, whose somatic concerns usually turn on contamination or rituals, the hypochondriac requires illness to maintain self-esteem and is voluble and querulous. The danger signs of depressive concern are those of lost self-esteem: illness is deserved, the patient is rejected because of it, no future is seen, the condition is terminal, and the presentation quiet and despairing, not aggressive and demanding. Any patient who believes his disease is incurable is more likely to be depressed than hypochondriacal. Sensitivity to this difference can be life saving.

It is necessary to agree that the hypochrondriac is ill, and to express surprise that, feeling so poorly, the patient is able to do so much (this judgment should be made reinforcing, not skeptical), and subsequent treatment is by the symbolic bottle of medicine, the scheduling of fixed appointments, and gradual reinforcement of alternative strategies. No threat is made to deprive such a patient of illness until this has been accomplished, although some hypochondriacal symptoms can be safely controlled by propranolol. If this schedule is mistakenly applied to a depressive, suicide will very probably occur. The hypochondriac's answer to questions about suicidal thoughts is pathognomonic by its aggressive manner. The depressed patient will either admit them quietly or avoid the question. The somatic concerns of the depressive should be met by reassurance (that no cancer is present, that he does not have syphilis) and simultaneously used to reinforce a strong suggestion that he accept hospital admission ("But you are obviously ill, and I think you should come into hospital"). If the physician does not have a talent for this sensitive balance, a psychiatric consult should be set up on an emergency basis. Depressed patients who are sent home to await admission or an appointment present a very high risk if depression is severe or deepens in the interval.

The hypochondriac is treatable and should be treated. Success in this operation calls for self-denial on the part of the doctor—not only in spending time, but in recognizing that the object of the exercise is to use the sickness—cure model implicit in office visits to a physician without threatening to cure the patient and thereby removing his or her security blanket. Progress is being made when sooner or later the patient stops blocking every interchange with a somatic complaint and begins to talk about such matters as anger, disappointment, and life failures. When this occurs a longer appointment should be scheduled and the patient listened to without interpretation. Often they themselves will interpret ("No wonder my head aches—it has been a pain in the neck"). Rather than leaping with relief on this admission, a therapist with good rapport will endorse it by facial expression, not with words. When this stage is reached, great benefit can come from group therapy, although it is important not to "shunt" the patient, thereby rejecting him; regular visits should continue. One can explain, "I really think it would help you now to discuss all these sad events in your life with other people; your own courage in dealing with them might be of help to people with similar problems." The day-attendance center is a particularly helpful venue for the old hypochondriac. It combines milieu therapy with the presence of a physician. The most resolute of career invalids are the first to take newcomers under their wing, with mutual benefit. In a more formal group, the hypochondriac is apt to backslide into discussing illness and will need protection from the initial irritation of group members. Good judgment is required to determine when a particular hypochondriacal patient is "ripe" to go public in this way.

"Psychopathic personalities," the chronically antisocial and maladjusted, tend to mellow with age. This clinical impression is supported by figures (Weiss, 1973), especially where the delinquent behavior was aggressive. The patient may have no more active a social conscience, but runs out of steam to express his defiance of society, and may agree better with society in consequence.

Bereavement is normally a response to the death or loss of a person, and as such, is increasingly common with increasing age, but it can also follow other losses—of a limb, of a pet, or of a beloved physical object. Its duration depends on the severity and significance of the loss, and it invariably includes a normal "work of mourning," which should not be medicated, harrassed with injunctions to look on the bright side, or boycotted, for it needs support. In severe bereavement, initial confusion, apathy, and denial are normal. The bereaved person may assert that, and act as if, the deceased person is alive. If this belief is made explicit by talking or writing letters to the lost one, it may be mistaken for pathology, which it is not. A special form of denial, closely similar to that of mourning, may be anosognosia, especially in stroke, where the illness itself is denied. Denial in whatever form may within two to three weeks give way to anger, then to a gradual and initially numb and unwilling resumption of customary activities, punctuated by sudden returns of acute grief when the loss is again brought to mind. In late life, where resilience is reduced, the stages of mourning may be prolonged, but few younger adults confronted with a serious loss complete them in less than six months to a year.

The treatment of grief is support, initially by being present and ensuring that essential measures (legal details, funeral arrangements) are conducted smoothly, and the bereaved protected from importunate condolence, frauds of all kinds, robbery by morticians, and attempts to "cheer them up." They should be encouraged to speak of the dead person, and to express feelings of guilt, loss, anger, or despair as these are experienced. Neither denial nor regression should be resisted by the therapist, nor should resumption of activities be insisted on until the bereaved is ready. If the geriatrician is the sole supporting person, daily sessions are indicated; the bereaved are commonly boycotted by their usual circle who "do not know what to say" to them. At the same time, vigilance for the transition from grief to depression, which takes place more easily in the old than in the young, must be exercised. Although bereaved people often say they do not want to go on living, suicide should be openly discussed if the patient expresses such ideas. Survivors of a long, mutually supporting marriage or friendship are exceptionally prone to see no means of remaking life. Overt, expressed grief is therapeutic; silence, insomnia, loss of weight and appetite, and undue duration of the normal stages of mourning require active intervention. Brief hospital care can sometimes prevent sorrow from passing into depressive illness and facilitate constructive regression. If severe depression does set in, it should be treated as an illness.

Reactive mania after bereavement is well documented (Rickarby, 1977; Hollinder and Goldin, 1978); it provides the factual base of the Victorian literary convention of madness from grief. In borderline patients mourning may be absent or of psychotic intensity. Minor or ingravescent bereavement is a common process of response to the losses of age—people who, though not very close to the patient, die one by one; skills, esteem, or futurity which are extinguished. In most old people, mourning is a component of ongoing experience which contains in miniature the features of major mourning and must be addressed in psychotherapy by recognition of its stages and giving support appropriate to each. For many of the old, loss is a way of life which must be experienced, addressed, and faced with the support of the physician as friend rather than as therapist.

Mr. H. was an 87-year-old immigrant of Russian extraction. He had formal schooling only until age 12, when he and his family entered the United States, but he was self-educated and of high intelligence and culture. Anxiety had long troubled him, and he was in receipt of an 80% service-connected disability pension for anxiety neurosis dating from World War I. For 58 years he had been married in what the notes termed "a coexistence relationship": His wife was a chronic invalid, and lately her illness had confined them to one another's company.

For two years Mr. H. had been becoming more depressed and withdrawn, and he had been hospitalized then for depression. Within a brief period he had encountered his wife's increasing disability, the death of his last surviving brother, a ticket for jaywalking which caused him much worry, and the closure of a neighborhood park where he and his friends used to meet. Under this combined pressure he had begun to drink heavily. Mr. H. had had a successful resection of prostatic and rectal carcinoma eight years previously, had a cardiac pacemaker inserted, and resection of his thyroid was performed during his last admission. While he was in hospital, his ailing wife died. Mr. H. reacted appropriately to this new loss. He moved to a Jewish home, but his feelings of isolation, guilt, rejection, and lack of concern for him on the part of his daughter and grandchildren, of whose successes he was deeply proud, were still painful. His drinking became an increasing problem, and his thoughts ran continually on death and suicide. After an anniversary reaction coinciding with Passover, he was readmitted.

Mr. H. was having ten separate medications (Esidrix, PGE, Aldomet, Librium, Tylenol, Darvon N, Urecholine, Anusol suppositories, and Metamucil), plus alcohol. Our function was to provide surrogate family support. Mr. H. was enabled to talk freely of his distress but was not urged to abreact; his stoicism was courage rather than denial. He had had attacks of nocturnal panic, which were traced to waking with a full bladder and being afraid of straining, which made him dyspneic and raised the fear that he would die as a result. Medication was reduced, his courage returned, and he controlled his drinking. Eventually he was able to return to the Jewish home with renewed fortitude, sad but not depressed. No psychoactive medication was necessary.

The management of bereavement in the old is an important preventive geriatric measure, deserving of considerable investment of time. A geriatric mental health center should be geared to give the necessary time and help, and must be publicly known to do so, so that others may call for assistance if the patient does not. Not only can such a service act to prevent major depressions, but at all ages relict spouses have an increased liability to unrelated disease and death as a direct result of their loss. Proper early care of the bereaved has, therefore, a preventive medical role. Death of a spouse is probably the most common indication for crisis intervention, and the team should have a strategy for such cases which meets the practical and emotional needs of the bereaved by supplying surrogate kin who act with knowledge.

Rehabilitation is not primarily "psychiatry" and is best done by those whose business it is—the rehabilitation teams of stroke, CVD, and orthopedic departments—provided that these exist, are effective, and recognize that the rehabilitative needs of the old exceed those of the young. Rehabilitation is required, moreover, in every geriatric patient whose illness is severe enough to require hospital admission. Where a geriatric unit admits stroke cases, in particular, the admission procedure should automatically alert the rehabilitation team so that it can begin work within 24 hours of the initial onset of illness. Waiting until patients "stabilize" or "recover function" after a stroke will seriously handicap their chances of regaining function at all (Adams, 1974).

GERIATRIC PSYCHIATRY AND THE LAW

Much of the geriatric psychiatrist's legal work will consist in testimony concerning guardianship, testamentary capacity, and mental competence. Guardianship proceedings which are resisted by the patient should go forward only if their subject is legally represented. The physician should decline to cooperate with informal proceedings, unless he or she is satisfied that the patient wishes them, and decline to provide reports to third parties. If subpoenaed, the physician should testify only under protest. A strong objection addressed to the court will, as a rule, lead to proper representation. Reports to attorneys or relatives made without patient consent constitute a breach of medical confidence. This may not be obvious under pressure, but it should be continually borne in mind.

At the same time, the value of voluntary guardianship should also be remembered. An old person who enters a hospital runs a risk of predation by neighbors and relatives, which can only be appreciated when it has been seen. Within hours of hospital admission, cars, apartments, and houses may have been sold, bearer bonds or jewelry appropriated, and even trifling effects looted by the loving and concerned entourage which has tended the old person and sees the opportunity for recompense. Theft of valuables, the holding of a free garage sale of the patient's effects, and the destruction of his home and means of transport can make discharge impossible, and the shock can cause permanent despair and death. Where the patient is able to consent, an early appointment of reliable counsel can nip this process of robbery in the bud, and it should be discussed with every old patient whose hospital stay is likely to exceed a few days. Where an active public guardian or public trustee exists, his office can and should be contacted. In other cases, a private attorney should be instructed. A geriatric assessment unit should maintain contacts for this purpose so that protection of property can be handled in appropriate cases as part of the admission procedure. This precaution is not one which needs to be reserved for the rich; no old persons, however limited their property, are safe from claim-jumping attacks on what they have if once they enter hospital, especially with a mental problem. This situation must be clearly distinguished from speculative guardianship proceedings instituted by relatives and may serve to forestall them.

The "Living Will" is likely to play an increasing part in geriatric practice. Euthanasia, in spite of some irrational advocacy, is not a serious issue. If depressives are excepted, it is what the relatives clamor for, rarely the patient. Patients who, faced with a prospect of painful illness and declining function, specifically seek death on realistic and considered grounds are surprisingly rare; far rarer than the situations which one might have expected to produce such a wish. Most are content to let nature take its course and accelerate that course only by ceasing to resist. In fact, if the patient has a sufficiently powerful will to die, death will indeed ensue, precisely as it can be held at bay in clinically unpromising circumstances by a sufficiently powerful short-term will to live, for example, to see a grandchild born or married, or to reach a landmark date or anniversary. The power of giving up is a resource which can sometimes be explained to the sick person who justifiably and realistically wishes to die. The obligation of the physician must be explained, firm reassurance must be given that pain can and will be controlled, and officious precautions against suicide must be avoided. The most important factor in alleviating such a situation is that patient and doctor talk frankly as friends and without playing games.

Far more often, reasonable people, including those still in good health, will have been found to have been upset by media reports of officious interference with the process of dying. Some of this anxiety is justified, but much of the propaganda which has generated it is based on ignorance, coupled with an Olympian failure on the part of physicians to make sure that patient and relatives understand what is being done, or may be done, and why. Some of the harm done by propaganda can be undone by frank discussion with patient and relatives of the medical bases on which treatment is given or withheld. They need to be told, first, that treatment which is more grievous than the disease and which offers no benefit will not be recommended, but that good medicine requires the relief of mental and physical suffering. Where complaint is made that a terminally ill person is receiving meddlesome or demeaning treatment, explanation is particularly in order—that the intravenous is designed to prevent suffering through dehydration and suction is designed to prevent distressing suffocation, and that nothing which is being done is part of an irrational attempt to prolong life regardless of its quality. To the anxious, dying patient, a firm guarantee that comfort will be maintained, pain controlled, and wishes respected is an important base for support and psychotherapy.

Mischief done by misstatement and misuse of the method is harder to undo in the case of ECT, since medical colleagues and formalities of approval reinforce the anxiety of an already gravely depressed patient. It can best be dealt with by a frank statement that this procedure is approximately as unpleasant to the patient as a dental extraction, that it will produce temporary confusion, that it is the only effective way of cutting short the misery he already feels, and that the consultant who has recommended it will administer it personally and remain present during recovery. In all these areas where public excitement and legal interference have created difficulties, the fault lies largely with failure of communication. They provide a model for all treatment decisions, however, for the surrender of autonomy implicit in becoming a patient is threatening as well as a reassuring reenactment of childhood needs. The physician who talks to patient and relatives and answers questions can retain the transference without reinforcing the threat.

Malpractice suits concerning the old are rarely based on genuine mistreatment, overmedication, or lack of geriatric training, which might properly provide a base for them; if they were, they would be far more common. They are more likely to be aimed at physicians whose proper and aggressive treatment of, for example, depression provokes a drug reaction or happens to coincide with an intercurrent embolism or heart attack. Although much malpractice litigation is commercial or vexatious in aim, this kind of suit may serve to cover large unconscious forces of next-of-kin guilt or denial of relief at the patient's death. The risk must be appreciated, but it cannot be allowed to dictate treatment. It may be necessary to explain forcefully to the court that depression is a life-threatening emergency and stand on the consciousness of responsibility to the patient without excessive looking over the shoulder.

The area of medical ethics, and of gauging responsibilities to the law and to the patient, is probably the only area of medical practice in which the physician has a professional duty to be arrogant. Obligatory and total amnesia in the face of demands for improper disclosure is an example. If this looks dangerous or uncivic, it is no more than the extension of the ultimate right of all citizens—"no laws are binding on the subject which assault the person or violate the conscience" (Blackstone). The problems of medical ethics do not, in fact, arise over the issues ("euthanasia," life support for vegetable patients) which convulse the media; in most cases, given the clinical situation, professional duty will be perfectly clear. Ethical problems far more often concern confidentiality and disclosure; they most commonly arise over what are not so much laws as regulations. This is particularly a problem in the United States, where officials are given to sweeping directives concerning such subjects as the use or nonuse of internationally accepted medications or the provision of confidential information for audit or statistical purposes. At any time, ethics may become an issue in geriatrics in the area of the allocation of resources—ineligibility of patients over a certain age for appropriate treatments such as surgery or dialysis on cost grounds. In all such matters, the best professional wisdom is that the doctor should obey scrupulously all major laws, ignore regulatory pettifogging of all kinds or conform with it nominally only, act on humane clinical judgment provided that he knows what he is doing, make diagnoses appropriate to frustrate nonmedical interference with treatment, and cultivate in all matters private and confidential to the patient a memory and a record system which, if improperly raided, are like the Bellman's map, a perfect and absolute blank. He will in such cases take the consequences if he must, but avoid them by foresight and subtlety if he can. The patient's welfare is his only concern, except in rare examples where others are seriously endangered.

SEXUALITY IN THE OLD

Human sexual needs and capacity are lifelong. A high proportion of older couples are, or are perfectly capable of being, sexually active, and aging itself is never a cause either of male impotence or of female incapacity (review: Comfort, 1978). Sexual dysfunction is, however, common at all ages. It is usually due to attitudinal conflict. When to the folklore of sex is added the folklore, and the real humiliations, of age, some people will use their age as an excuse to unload an anxiety-provoking function. Others will succumb to social pressure. Yet others, chiefly women, to whom social mythology is especially cruel, may experience loss of opportunity and react with resignation and role playing. Some old people find either capacity or opportunity compromised by age-associated causes (medication, surgery, bereavement) and react with extreme disturbance over the loss, but do not volunteer it. Yet others, having experienced loss or castration in the area of social roles and self-value, undergo a secondary loss of sexual capacity, which reflects their diminished sense of gender identity.

Common remediable problems in previously functioning old people are (a) erectile difficulties due to performance anxiety, medication, diabetes, undiagnosed Peyronie's disease, or problems of or with the partner: these call for proper investigation, specific treatment, and counseling and education in all cases from all causes; (b) anatomical problems in women—prolapse, cystocele, dryness and dyspareunia, and cosmetic changes such as pendulous breasts which affect morale of either partner: these call for judicious surgical repair, exercises, or local estrogens; and (c) anhedonia, which may reflect physical illness, giving up, or, very commonly, undiagnosed depression, of which it is an important sign. Vigorous attempts to preserve continued sexual function, to suggest alternative strategies where there is disability, and to neutralize folklore by encouragement are always worthwhile. Most males are ignorant of the normal age changes toward a need for stronger penile stimulation and less regular ejaculation at every act. Systemic estrogens are best avoided—systemic androgens are of limited use only, chiefly in improving well being: the best resources are treatment of disability and encouragement by reassurance.

Sexual problems should be tactfully included in all geriatric psychiatric histories. They are no less present than in youth, only less often inquired for, and they may play a large part in triggering insomnia, depression, or the general syndrome of loss and despair. Sexual counseling is especially necessary in the psychiatric work of rehabilitation after illness and in minimizing the effects of surgery (prostatectomy, hysterectomy) which can induce sexual dysfunction not only by physical changes but also by bewitchment through thoughtlessly prohibitive or insufficiently explicit and reassuring advice. With the advent of sleep phallometry, it is no longer necessary to rely on anecdotal evidence to diagnose psychogenic impotence (Karacan, 1978). Sexual dysfunction in the old is not so often referred to the psychiatrist as at younger ages, but a diligent questioner will often uncover it. Organic precipitants such as drug effects, obesity, alcohol, and CNS disease should be sought and couple therapy instituted exactly as with the young. Although many old people received their sexual education and style 50 years ago, many appreciate and are relieved by the opportunity to discuss now experiences and needs which could not decently be discussed before. In residential homes, retirement communities, and group sessions, sexuality is a topic which, once introduced, produces much relief. Patients who prefer not to explore the matter will usually make their wishes clear, and these wishes should be respected.

With the growing attitude of sexual openness in society, little has been done to preserve function in the old. Staff must be educated not to treat normal appetency as evidence of senility. Separation of married couples in institutions should be seen as an outrage, which it is. Patronizing and childrenizing solutions, which seem to appeal particularly to the rigidly institution minded—petting rooms, permission to hold hands under close chaperonage, mockery or sedation of older men and women who wish to marry or who contract affairs—need replacing with dignity. The old who through no fault of their own are forced to live under the supervision of others are entitled to the same freedom in personal relations as they would enjoy at home, subject only to common sense precautions against harrassment or scandal to weaker brethren. For the old spouse in hospital and for the dying, conjugal visits are perhaps more important than at younger ages. Disuse threatens function, deprivation causes loss of self-esteem, and death requires sexual leave taking. In these matters, the physician can act with frankness, communication, and understanding without appearing to intrude. Reassurance over masturbation is necessary in both sexes (Feigenbaum, 1974) and at all ages. Problems of gender identity are not outlived; homosexual anxieties which surface in age need not be sought at the depth level, but they can be addressed and often healed by discussion when conscious. Sexuality has greatly different meanings for different people—it may be unimportant, a consuming preoccupation, a leading source of self-validation, a major focus of anxiety, or a continual solace (sometimes more than one of these). Sometimes in the geriatric period insight is more easily gained into such matters than it would have been in youth, given permission and opportunity without impertinent pressure.

Problems with anxious staff are becoming less common; they have also changed in form with the sexual climate and are no longer expressed in moralistic terms. Occasionally, it must be pointed out that a sexually appetent individual who is isolated will masturbate, that lacking privacy such an individual may masturbate coram publico, and that a depressed or pain-afflicted patient may well masturbate frequently, taking advantage of the transient antidepressant and analgesic effects of orgasm. These considerations are "geriatric" only in that the old are most subjected, with the disabled, to loss of privacy and scrutiny by others.

A 67-year-old man with bulbar palsy and urinary infection was desolated by the loss of his wife. In hospital, despite a Foley catheter, he masturbated four or five times a day, using shaving cream as a lubricant and scattering it about the ward bathroom. Concern was expressed at the risk of self-injury. It was represented to the staff that the patient was lucky to retain this resource in the ruin of his world, and that the consultant would hope to be able to do the same, given similar circumstances. The patient was counseled to the same effect, while directing his attention to Mrs. Patrick Campbell's advice against "doing it in the street and frightening the horses," which produced his first smile since his admission.

8

A GERIATRIC
MENTAL HEALTH
SERVICE

MENTAL HEALTH CARE

The delivery of mental health care in old age is a function of health care delivery in general, national ideology, and degree of commitment to the welfare of older people. It presents a problem to all countries, given the increase in survival to high ages and the changes in family structure which are now universal in the developed world, but some countries have more integrated and more successful systems than others. In general, these tend to be countries where a community-based structure of long standing, originating in the village, has been translated into modern terms, where health is regarded as a service rather than sickness as an industry, and where large population movements and high mobility are absent.

The value of experience derived from Britain, Scandinavia, the major Euro-powers, and Canada for the American psychogeriatrician is less as a political model than as a source of guidelines for what can and should be delivered. The attitude toward self and sources of value of older people and the style of political organization are deeply rooted in national styles. Rather than approach the welfare of patients and the prerequisites for good medical practice on a basis of ideological commitment to "national health care" or commercial laissez-faire, the pragmatic approach would seem to be to examine what is needed, using the experience of geriatrically advanced countries, and to contrast it with what is not being done. The second of these has been sharply documented (Butler, 1975), but the first has barely been addressed.

British experience indicates, on a basis of practical trial, that the most effective deliverer of primary geriatric care in all areas is the family practitioner. In Europe, he is familiar with his patients and makes house calls, which are essential in geriatric practice. He may operate alone or in partnership. In the case of group practice operating from a neighborhood health center, one physician will commonly concentrate on geriatric medicine and the team will have the support of social workers and close liaison with integrated local authority services (housing, home nursing, social security), which are integral to and form part of any effective system of senior health care. The second line of service is the hospital geriatric department operating as a point of referral and staffed by a specialist geriatrician. For each major population center, one geriatric hospital department, preferably in a teaching hospital, operates as a geriatric psychiatric assessment center. The assignment of such a center is to diagnose difficult cases, including the investigation of psychosis and dementia, to screen out secondary or iatrogenic mental illness, and to schedule treatment and rehabilitation programs for referral back to the responsible physician—either the family practitioner or the medical officer of an institution. A center of this kind requires the services of a psychiatrist, internist, psychopharmacologist, and clinical psychologist with a full range of consult facilities and the ability to conduct complete work-ups, perform medical and neurological tests at a sophisticated level, and operate at high turnover, discharging patients to other facilities after diagnosis. Where a psychodiagnostic center forms part of the geriatric department of a teaching hospital, it will play an important part in training future physicians and surgeons of all specialties during their clinical course, under a professor of geriatric medicine. Both teaching and local hospitals will operate high-turnover geriatric wards with discharge either to the patient's home, with in-home support services provided by the local authority, or to home supplemented by a day attendance center, or to a residential institution.

Day attendance centers are not confined to psychiatric patients, to the very infirm, or to patients under treatment. Although they can provide facilities and treatment for all geriatric patients in need of support (Table 8.1), they also function as clubs and social centers for the ambulatory old, meals centers, and monitoring points which relieve the load on primary care physicians, institutions, and relatives. They are particularly important for implementation of the principle that in older people, institutionalization should be avoided as bedrest is avoided. Day attendance centers are both more effective and more cost-effective than custodial "homes." They are not specifically psychiatric, since they include all forms of rehabilitation, including fracture and stroke, and well patients, but they serve a general psychotherapeutic function in enriching environment, breaking down loneliness, and providing settings for group discussion, including therapy and social groups. A day attendance center must have transport to bring in patients and a "chaser" equipped with a vehicle to check on defaulters. Some of these will be ill and require medical attention; others may merely be held back by minor obstacles such as loss of a button which they are unable to replace unaided. Because defaulters readily drop out of the program, all of them require to be "chased." Patients from

TABLE 8.1. Procedures Appropriate to Day Hospital

Intraarticular injections	Bladder wash-outs
Weekly blood tests	ECT
(e.g., patients on anticoagulants)	Physiotherapy
Electrocardiogram	Occupational therapy
Sigmoidoscopy	Rehabilitation
Glucose tolerance test	Group psychotherapy
Test meal	Relatives' support groups
Marrow puncture	Sexual and family counseling
Lumbar puncture	Bereavement support
Aspirations	Hospice program
Blood transfusion	Legal clinic
Intravenous total dose iron therapy	Meals service
Catheterization	"Enrichment": tours, visits, events

From Strouthidis, T.M. (1974).

nursing homes can attend the day center, thereby providing occupational opportunities and variety, which are difficult for a small institution to provide, plus a continual check on status and medication.

THE PSYCHOGERIATRIC ASSESSMENT CENTER

A psychogeriatric ward is an acute ward. It should have no provision for custodial cases or for long-stay "graduates." This is of paramount importance. "Traditionally, an admission ward is an area where nursing and other staff have high expectations for patients and are much involved with them. Too often in psychogeriatric wards the staff are so busy with the general care of their handicapped patients that direct stimulation of patients tends to go by the board" (Thomson, 1977). Under no circumstances should "diagnostic beds" be put in a custodial psychogeriatric ward. If the assessment unit is confined to a few beds, they should form part of a general admission unit, including adults and adolescents. In Thomson's unit, 64% of those with senile dementias admitted to the acute ward and 23.5% of similar patients admitted to the psychogeriatric (custodial) ward were discharged from hospital. The disadvantage (of further limiting the population of the psychogeriatric ward to "hopeless cases") may be offset by the advantages of selecting and training special staff for long-term care functions if these are to be undertaken.

Initial examination is by the geriatric internist as well as the psychiatrist, if these are different individuals. Between 50 and 70% of admissions to such a unit will have immediate problems of overt disease, diagnosis, or medication. Using European diagnostic criteria, between 33 and 50% of the admissions will be for investigation of acute or ingravescent intellectual impairment, about 25% will have primarily affective symptoms, and about 5% will have diagnoses related to schizophrenia. Other problems will include crisis interventions, alcoholism, and neuropsychiatric problems.

The psychodiagnostic unit must have an extramural capability. In many cases, initial case taking may have to be done in the home; after discharge, extramural nurses play an important part in reducing hospital admission (Prinsley, 1978), and it is hard to see how an effective noncustodial unit can be maintained without them, unless all patients are discharged to day centers. In-home support facilities represent the difference between continued domiciliary life and needless hospital admission. In some cases, the "flying squad" will act as a crisis unit; in most cases, its function will be diagnostic.

Outpatients and the custodial or long-term ward, if there is one, should come under the sovereignty of the admission unit: the first, to enable integration of initial treatment with follow-up; the second to ensure constant re-evaluation. Although some patients should be in long-term care and should not be disturbed, length of time in hospital before the creation of an aggressive diagnostic and rehabilitation program is no index of unsuitability for discharge. A shakeout is normal in the "chronic" ward when such a unit comes into existence. It occurs in two waves: one of revised diagnoses, and the second through the introduction of trained rehabilitation social workers who can make the necessary arrangements and carry them through. At the same time, the physician in charge of long-term care should be a generalist who also has acute beds; the geriatric specialist whose only charges are long-term patients is easily extruded from general medicine.

Medical students and student nurses should be assigned not only to the acute admission and evaluation ward but also to outpatients and to long-term care. Nothing does more to break down defeatism that to see the first, and nothing does more to inculcate concern and realism than the second.

Old people may be more stoical, less likely to identify their complaints as curable, and more scared of psychiatry and of hospitals than young patients, but when psychiatric services which they can reach and afford are provided, they make use of them, with therapeutic results very similar to those in the young (Feigenbaum, 1974). The main complaints presenting to such a service, where it is provided, will be depressive. Drug problems, including alcohol, but with a preponderance of prescribed overmedication, and sexual problems, will be frequent. Feigenbaum's elderly patient who had received 12 different psychoactive drugs in two months, and was demented in consequence, is by no means atypical of the first type of problem. Strong sexual feelings in elderly women brought up to feel guilty about them, worry over masturbation, and depression following impotence or the impotence of a spouse are typical of the second. Geriatric psychiatry which sees itself as geared to dealing with senile dementia and uninvolved in active psychotherapy will be quite unable to tackle the reality. For this reason, psychiatric assessment centers must provide exactly the same services and referrals for human problems, educational forms of therapy such as sex counseling and counseling in the realities of aging, group therapy, and prescribing as any general mental health service. Correct diagnosis of supposed "senile" illness will be important, but most of the cases found to be remediable will need access to standard forms of treatment, modified only by the need for additional support against society's assaults on the older citizen. This should be made clear to staff in the initial training and selection process; they will be working in general mental health secundum artem, not in custodial nursing.

A STRATEGY FOR GERIATRIC PSYCHIATRY IN AMERICA

A comprehensive system of geriatric mental health which involves university departments, statutory agencies, local facilities, and the physician's own practice is beyond the capacity of the individual practitioner to organize. On the other hand, since it may well prove that the optimal American model of health care delivery is local in emphasis, the staff of health maintainance organizations, hospitals, and geriatric institutions can produce programs which address both patient needs and the overriding need to create demonstrations of good geriatric psychiatry in practice.

One logical model would be to combine a psychiatric assessment center with a day attendance center. Day centers are by common consent of experience best located in a hospital (Strouthidis, 1974) to avoid duplication of staff and facilities. If space is set apart, they can well be associated with a psychogeriatric assessment ward. In fact, where a psychogeriatric ward is conducted in conjunction with outpatients and is accessible, an informal day center commonly comes into existence, composed of discharged patients returning for check up, for medication, or to visit inpatients. It becomes more practical to organize space for these incomers than to have them waiting on benches or sitting in the day rooms.

The most common, if unspoken, objection to a designated psychodiagnostic unit, which causes hospital administrators or physicians to say that it is "not needed," is the fear that it will generate chronic bed occupancy and become "clogged." The coexistence of a day program is a strong guarantee of high turnover, and it can be funded in terms of the saving of bed space. Most of its activities can be piggybacked on already existing occupational, medical, or rehabilitation facilities, with some gain, in that admixture with young, nonpsychiatric patients is achieved. Recovering patients can (and should) be given occupational responsibility as volunteers in a therapeutic community model. Where difficulty arises over cost of transport, local volunteer and senior organizations—and in some cases the school district, which may have idle buses and staff during day hours—can be involved. In this way, a functioning psychogeriatric unit can with determination and financial persuasiveness be created on a grassroots basis by accretion. Arguments based on lowering the overall cost of service and reduction of wasteful hospital admission are extremely effective in dealing with formalistic and territorial disputes. The creation of a day center program is not beyond the resources of an HMO or a physician group if it has community support and available volunteers. Such a center may not be able to provide all the services available in a hospital, but it can provide some of them. A day hospital program, moreover, rapidly acquires a constituency, both from seniors and from physicians and relatives relieved by its existence, which can apply political pressure to secure subvention and outface administrative rigidity.

A direct-action model of this kind tends to operate by improvization to meet local conditions, but it can and should study published experience (Irvine, 1974). For example, if transport is to be purchased, rather than available vehicles borrowed, it should be suitable. Ambulances in which elderly people are crowded without being able to see out are unsuitable and aggravate confusion and disorientation (Hildick-Smith, 1974); minibuses produce difficulties of access and are "half-suitable."

Although day care spares hospital beds, it functions chiefly as a supplement to long-term care rather than as a substitute for short-term admission to the ward. Many day-care patients are eventually admitted as a result of growing infirmity, while others become dependent on the day center as a support mechanism and will have to be admitted if the day program closes (Arie, 1975). Very confused patients benefit little because of the added confusion due to travel and the fact that, having forgotten each week what happened in the previous week, the arrangement needs constant renegotiation. Isolated, hypochondriacal, and clinic-dependent people, so far from being querulous and unbenefited "trolls," provide a continuity to the program by acting as anchors and by hosting new entrants to their mutual benefit. Most of these would have occupied the time of physicians rather than hospital beds, but their diversion into day programs is extremely cost-effective in cutting down on unnecessary office visits. Reorganization of the nursing-home centered care system into lodging care and day attendance could greatly reduce both its cost and its present inefficacy while upgrading its standards by regular medical supervision of long-term patients.

THE EDUCATION OF GERIATRICIANS

The most urgent problem in American geriatrics is training. The United States has one professorship of geriatric medicine as opposed to 14 in the United Kingdom, and no professorship of geriatric psychiatry. Excellent research is undertaken in basic science, certain medical schools have good postgraduate programs, and the Veterans Administration and the great Jewish hospitals both have considerable commitments to clinical teaching. The fact remains, however, that geriatrics in general is otherwise not taught, that centers of excellence are few, and that growing demographic pressure suggests an ominous future in which, after a multiplication of self-appointed "geriatric" and "geriatric psychiatric" specialists, staff will be headhunted from European and Canadian programs to handle the demand. Even if outsiders were recruited, the possibility of general indoctrination with geriatrics in family practice up to European standards (Caird, 1978) seems remote.

A training program for cadres, including fellowships similar to those now offered by the Veterans Administration, coupled with exchange fellowships,

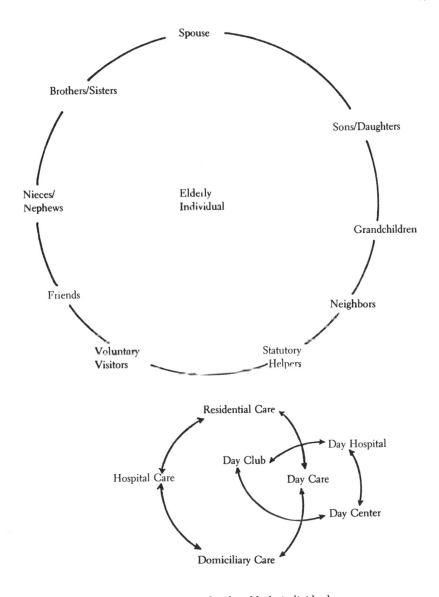

FIGURE 8.1. Community resources for the elderly individual.
From Hall, M.R.P. *In* Irvine, R.F., (1974).

could create a body of teachers which would make it possible to incorporate geriatrics in the general medical curriculum (and reduce the burden on specialist geropsychiatry by improving diagnosis, prescribing, and management). No single reform would be more beneficial than the inclusion of geriatric questions in the medical licensure examinations.

Since geriatric patients will account for about 60% of office practice in the next few years, and psychiatric problems for perhaps 25% of that, instruction in geriatrics and geriatric psychiatry would seem a reasonable requirement for all physicians now in training who will not be neonatologists or pediatricians.

Unfortunately, this is not what is happening. Instead, we see a proliferation of courses in "social gerontology" catering to young persons who formerly "wanted to teach" but now, education having run out of public credit, "want to work with the old." We see courses in leisure organization, courses in lecturing to old people, the steady creation of a vast geroparasitic organization, all of which will have to be fed, and intends to live off the country. Far too many programs have gone this way in the past. For every $100 set aside by Congress or by the states to aid a social problem, we have come to fear, if not to expect, that $50 will go in "preliminary studies" and $40 in other forms of welfare for administrative and helping personnel. The training of career "grannyologists" as a substitute for the development of proper services has become an activity of several academic centers and has resulted in a flood of literature which is poor even by the standards of social science, while the growth of a granny industry threatens to produce a boondoggle proportionate to the demographic increase in the host animal, the older American.

This need not be. Academic centers, and particularly teaching hospitals, can develop geriatric psychiatry as a normal feature of medical education (not as a source of additional specialists) and local medicine can develop its implementation. But both these developments depend on attitudinal change. Medicine and psychiatry might wish to see them for strictly professional reasons, but they are also a necessary part of what might be termed "holistic citizenship." If we do not want to see our dollars wasted, we can enlist parsimony in the cause of principle. What matters is that the psychiatric services available to the old shall not continue to lag behind the state of world knowledge and the state of practice in other civilized countries.

Ideological in-fighting over methods of funding health care can only delay this desirable result and render patients disgruntled with the profession. If physicians quite reasonably fear bureaucratization, either by government or by commercial insurers, they have to hand the traditional remedy of direct action—namely, creating local institutions with the cooperation of patients, of senior citizen advocacy groups, and of the community. For such an initiative, there is already a massive constituency.

COURSE IN GERIATRIC PSYCHIATRY
proposed for
Veterans Administration Geriatric Fellows 1979

Clinical geriatric Fellows are well-qualified (usually Board certified) physicians of considerable experience. The object of this draft curriculum, which is the sole responsibility of the author, not of the Veterans Administration, is to outline what they should be prepared to teach, given that their role will be as future professors of geriatric medicine. It is included here as a suggested model for what all courses in geriatric psychiatry should be prepared to teach.

1. Introductory. Biological gerontology and the nature of physical aging.
2. Psychometrics of normal aging: learning, intelligence, adaptation.
3. The experience of aging. Life cycle: change in role identity; loss versus ego-integrity; present vs. futurity; posterity; death.
4. The experience of aging in America. Agism: retirement; dependency and the stereotype of independence; effects of changes in family structure; the "new old," agism, racism, and minorities. Society and self-valuation.
5. The physician as geriatric psychiatrist—overview: basic concepts of geriatrics; physical causes of mental symptoms; common psychiatric problems of the old.
6. The physician as geriatric psychiatrist: differential diagnosis of "senility"; failure to thrive in the senium.
7. Physical disorders presenting as confusion. Iatrogenic mental disorder.
8. Psychoses in age. Affective disorder: diagnosis and treatment.
9. Psychoses in age. Schizophrenia. Differential diagnosis, schizoaffective illnesses, late paraphrenia.
10. Psychoses in age. Paranoia as a nonspecific symptom. Sensory deficit paranoias. Paranoid psychoses.
11. Neurosis in age: panic states; hypochondriasis; old age of the chronic neurotic; anxiety and its management.

12. Psychopharmacology of old age. Therapeutic and adverse effects of general and of psychoactive drugs.

13. Dementia. Organic causes; Alzheimer; thromboembolic dementia; alcoholic dementia; other organic causes.

14. Differential diagnosis of the dementias; investigations; psychometric testing.

15. Treatment and management of dementias; experimental drugs; reality therapy; institutional vs. home; day hospitals; role of psychodiagnostic unit.

16. Psychometric testing and tests in geriatric practice.

17. Psychotherapy with the old; uses of support; historical vs. supportive and existential models; group therapy; nature of transference and countertransferences.

18. Countertransference and physician insight; reason the old threaten the physician; counseling with staff and family members.

19. The old person in the family: conflicts; denial; guilt; dependency; the abused older person.

20. Nursing homes and institutions: as they are and as they could be; role of the geriatric consultant; staff training; models.

21. Poverty, entitlement, and social services in America.

22. Role and functions of the geriatric social worker; in-home support of the old.

23. In-home, community, and institutional models of care delivery. The family practitioner; European and Canadian models of geriatric care. Day centers, outreach.

24. Legal implications of geriatric practice. Testamentary capacity, guardianship, predation by relatives, meddlesome therapy in terminal illness, protection of the geriatric patient.

25. Terminal illness. The approach of death in early vs. late life. Family therapy. Group therapy. The hospice model.

26. Geriatric care problems: the expertise of the nurse; support, family-surrogation; special problems (decubitus ulcers, confusion, wandering).

27. The geriatric team: physician, nurse, psychologist, social worker. Insight and interaction.

28. Sleep, its disorders, and their management in the senium.

29. Alcoholism and addiction to medication in old age.

30. Special problems of psychiatric treatment: coexistent heart disease; mobility difficulties; diabetes; arthritis; sensory deficits.

31. Normal and abnormal sexuality in later life: function and dysfunction; impotency and its investigation; the older deprived woman; institutional problems.

32. Education in old age; "discovery" programs; SAGE and the California smörgasbord; psychodrama, art, creativity.

33. Prospective counseling: driving ability, mobility, housing for the old, income planning, physician-assisted foresight.

34. The utopian "geriatric service": what do we want, how can it be obtained, what will be its mental-health aspects?

35. Crisis intervention: house moving, bereavement, suicide, acting-out crises, acute confusion, self-neglect.

36. Religious and philosophical aspects of age: the concept of samnyasa; the old as elders; oceanic experiences and the linearity of time; religious traditions; relevance to patient experience.

NOTES

The course is angled to graduate physicians, but its material will be presented as relevant to all geriatric team members.

Edification will be implicit, not sententious; the lecturers should be role models.

Opportunity should be given for entrants to discuss in group their own feelings and attitudes to aging and the old with psychiatric leadership.

Every outline presentation should be (a) accompanied by a reading list, (b) illustrated by additional case presentations, and (c) linked to back-up specialist lectures and workshops amplifying specific therapeutic, nursing, or other techniques.

Administrative who-does-what and similar chinoiseries should be subordinated to the object of the course, which is to benefit patients and to prepare us to benefit them, not to minister to our own unconscious needs. Where these needs conflict with the aims of the course, we should attempt to obtain insight into them.

REFERENCES

Abrams, R. (1979) The ECT controversy: Observations and a suggestion. Psychiatr. Opinion 16.11–15.

Abrams, R. and Taylor, M. (1976) Catatonia: A prospective clinical study. Arch. Gen. Psychiatry 33:579–581.

Adams, G.F. (1974) Cerebrovascular Disorder and the Ageing Brain. Edinburgh, Churchill-Livingstone.

Appelbaum, P.S., Vasile, R.G., Orsulak, P.J., and Schildkraut, J.J. (1979) Clinical utility of tricyclic antidepressant blood levels: A case report. Am. J. Psychiatry 136:339–340.

Ashley, M.I., Olin, J.S., le Riche, W.H., Kornaczewski, A., Schmidt, W., and Rankin, J.G. (1976) Continuous and intermittent alcoholics. Addict. Dis. 2:515–532.

Bahemuka, M. and Hodkinson, H.M. (1975) Screening for hypothyroidism in elderly patients. Br. Med. J. 2:601–603.

Barker, J.L. (1976) Peptides: Roles in neuronal excitability. Physiol. Rev. 56:435–448.

Bartter, F. and Schwartz, W.B. (1976) The syndrome of inappropriate secretion of antidiuretic hormone. Am. J. Med. 49:790–806.

Beckmann, H. and Goodwin, F.K. (1975) Antidepressant response to tricyclics and urinary MHPG in unipolar patients. Arch. Gen. Psychiatry 32:17–20.

Bennett, J.P., Arregui, A., and Snyder, S.H. (1976) Angiotensin II as a possible mammalian neurotransmitter. Abstract presented at the 6th Annual Meeting of the Society of Neurosciences, Toronto, p. 775.

Bergmann, K. (1978) Neurosis and personality disorder in old age. In Isaacs, A.D. and Post, F. Studies in Geriatric Psychiatry. Chichester, John Wiley.

Bethune, H.C., Burrell, R.H., Culpan, R.H. and Ogg, G.J. (1964) Vascular crises associated with MAOIs. Am. J. Psychiatry 3:245–253.

Birkett, D.P. (1971) Cerebral vasodilators. Br. Med. J. 4:235.

Blessed, G., Tomlinson B.E., and Roth M. (1968) Evaluation of a mental test score for assessment of mental impairment in the elderly. Br. J. Psychiatry 114:797–804.

Bleuler, M. (1972) Die Schizophrenen Geistesstörungen. Stuttgart, Georg Thieme.

Bowen, D.M. (1977) Biochemistry of dementias. Proc. R. Soc. Med. 70:351–352.

Bowen, D.M. (1978) Biochemical changes in the normal aging brain. In Isaacs, B. (ed) Recent Advances in Geriatric Medicine. Vol. I. New York, Churchill-Livingstone.

Bowen, D.M., Smith, C.B., White, P., Goodhardt, M.J., Spillane, J.A., Flack, R.H.A., and Davison, A.N. (1977a) Chemical pathology of the organic dementias, I. Brain 100:397–426.

Bowen D.M., Smith C.B., White P., Flack R.H.A., Carrasco L., Gedye, J.L., and Davison, A.N. (1977b) Chemical pathology of the organic dementias, II. Brain 100:427–454.

Boyd, R.V. and Woodman, J.A. (1978) The Jekyll-and-Hyde syndrome. Lancet ii:671–672.

Boyd, W.D., Graham-White, J., Blackwood, G., Glen, I., and McQueen, J. (1977) Clinical effects of choline in Alzheimer senile dementia. Lancet ii:711.

Brewer, C. and Perrett, L. (1971) Brain damage due to alcohol consumption. Br. J. Addict. 66:170–182.

Brook, P., Degren, G., and Mather, M. (1975) Reality orientation—a therapy for psychogeriatric patients. Br. J. Psychol. 127:42–45.

Brown, G.W., Bhrolchain, M.N., and Harris, T. (1975) Social class and psychiatric disturbance among women in an urban population. Sociology 9:225–254.

Brinkley, J.R., Beitman, B.D., and Friedel, R.O. (1979) Low-dose neuroleptic regimens in the treatment of borderline patients. Arch. Gen. Psychiatry 36:319–326.

Butler, R.N. (1975) Why survive? Growing Old in America. New York, Harper and Row.

Caird, F.I. (1978) The state of British medicine: The teaching of geriatrics. J. R. Soc. Med. 71:711–715.

Carlson, G.A. and Goodwin, F.K. (1973) The stages of mania—a longitudinal analysis of the manic episode. Arch. Gen. Psychiatry 28:221–228.

Cavenar, J.O., Sullivan, J.L., and Maltbie, A.A. (1979) A clinical note on hysterical psychosis. Am. J. Psychiatry 136:830–832.

Charney, D.S. (1979) Sleep architecture in psychotropic-induced somnambulism. Am. J. Psychiatry 136:461.

Chien, C.P., Stotsky, B.A., and Cole, J.O. (1973) Psychiatric treatment for nursing-home patients: Drug, alcohol and milieu. Am. J. Psychiatry 130:543–548.

Clarke, J. and Haughton, H. (1975) A study of intellectual impairment and recovery rates in heavy drinkers in Ireland. Br. J. Psychiatry 126:178–184.

Comfort, A. (1978) Drug therapy in Alzheimer's disease. Lancet i:659.

Comfort, A. (ed) (1978) Sexual Consequences of Disability. Philadelphia, Geo. Stickley Co.

Coppen, A. Shaw, D.M., Herzberg, B., and Maggs, R. (1967) Tryptophan in the treatment of depression. Lancet ii 1178–1180.

Coppen, A., Noguera, R., Bailey, J., Burns, B. H., Swani, M.S., Hare, H., Gardner, R., and Maggs, R. (1971) Prophylactic lithium in affective disorders. Lancet ii:275–279.

Coppen, A., Ghose, K., Rao, R., Bailey, J., and Peet, M. (1978) Mianserin and lithium in the prophylaxis of depression. Br. J. Psychiatry 133:206–210.

Corsellis, J.A.N. (1962) Mental illness and the aging brain. London, Oxford University Press.

Crapper, D.R., Krishan, S.S., and Dalton, A.J. (1973) Brain aluminum distribution in Alzheimer's disease and experimental neurofibrillary degeneration. Science 180:511–513.

D'Alarcon, R. (1964) Hypochondriasis and depression in the aged. Gerontol. Clin. (Basel) 6:266–277.

Davies, P. and Maloney, A.J.F. (1976) Selective loss of central cholinergic neurons in Alzheimer's disease. Lancet ii:1403.

Davison, A.N. (1977) Chemical pathology of brain degeneration. Proc. R. Soc. Med. 70:349–350.

Davison, K. (1964) Episodic depersonalisation: observations on seven patients. Br. J. Psychiatry 110:505–513.

Dekoninck, W.J., Collard M., and Noel, S. (1977) Cerebral vasoactivity in senile dementia. Gerontology 23:148–160.

Denham, M.J. and Jeffrys, P.M. (1972) Routine mental assessment of elderly patients. Mod. Geriatr. 2:275–279.

Drachman, D.A. (1974) Human memory and the cholinergic system. Arch. Neurol. 30.113–121.

Dunleavy, D.L.F. and Oswald, I. (1973) Phenelzine, mood response and sleep. Arch. Gen. Psychiatry 28:353–356.

Eichhorn, O. (1965) The effect of cyclandelate on cerebral circulation. Vasc. Dis. 2:305–310.

Eisdorfer, C., Nowlin, J., and Wilkie F. (1970). Improvement of learning in the aged by modification of autonomic nervous system activity. Science 170:1327–1329.

Ernst, K. (1959) Die Prognose der Neurosen. Monogr. Neurol. Psychiatry 85: Berlin, Springer Verlag.

Ernst, P., Badash, D., Beran B., Kosovsky, R., and Kleinhaus, M. (1977) Psychiatric problems of the aged. J. Am. Geriatr. Soc. 25:371–375.

Evans, B.V. (1970) Thyroid hormone and tricyclic antidepressants in resistant depressions. Am. J. Psychiatry 126:1667–1669.

Feigenbaum, E.M. (1974) Geriatric psychopathology—internal or external? J. Am. Geriatr. Soc. 22:49–56.

Finch, C.E. (1976) The regulation of physical changes during mammalian aging. Rev. Biol. 51:49–83.

Folsom, J.C. (1968) Reality orientation therapy. J. Geriatr. Psychiatry 1:291–307.

Forbes, A. (1949) Dream scintillations. Psychosom. Med. 2:160–163.

Foster, J.R., Gershell W.J., and Goldfarb, A.I. (1977) Lithium treatment for the elderly. I. Clinical usage. J. Gerontol. 32:299–302.

Fox, J.H., Topel, J.L., and Huckman, M.S. (1975) Use of computerized tomography in senile dementia. J. Neurol. Neurosurg. Psychiatr. 38:948–953.

Fraser, R.M. and Glass, I.B. (1978) Recovery from ECT in elderly patients. Br. J. Psychiatry 133:524–528.

Freedman, R. and Schwab, P.J. (1978) Paranoid symptoms in patients on a general hospital psychiatric unit. Arch. Gen. Psychiatry 35:387–390.

Fry, D.E. and Marks, V. (1971) Value of plasma lithium monitoring. Lancet i:886–888.

Gaitz, C.M., Varner, R.V., and Overall, J.E. (1977) Pharmacotherapy for organic brain syndrome in late life. Arch. Gen. Psychiatry 34:839–842.

Gaitz, C.M. and Baer, P.E. (1971) Characteristics of elderly patients with alcoholism. Arch. Gen. Psychiatry 24:372–378.

Gajdusek, D.C. (1974) Slow and latent viruses in the aged nervous system. *In* Maletta, G.J. Survey Report on the Aging Nervous System. DHEW NIH 74–296, pp. 149–162.

Gajdusek, D.C., Gibbs, C.I., Asher, D.M., Brown, P., Diwan, A., Hoffman, P., Nemo, G., Rohwer, R., and White, L. (1977) Precautions in the medical care of patients with Creutzfeldt–Jakob Disease. N. Engl. J. Med. 297:1264–1267.

Gedye, J.L., Exton-Smith, A.N., and Wedgwood, J. (1972) A method for measuring mental performance in elderly patients and its use in a pilot clinical trial of mec-lofenoxate in organic dementia. Age and Aging 1:74–80.

Gilmore, A.J.J. (1972) Personality in the elderly: Problems of methodology. Age and Aging 4:227–232.

Goldfarb, A.L. (1971) Geropsychiatry in the general hospital. Mt. Sinai J. Med. 38:79–88.

Gosling, R.H. (1955) The association of dementia with radiologically demonstrated cerebral atrophy. J. Neurol. Neurosurg. Psychiatry 18:129–133.

Grant, I. and Mohns, L. (1975) Chronic cerebral effects of alcohol and drug abuse. Int. J. Addict. 10:883–920.

Hachinski, V.C., Lassen, N.A., and Marshall, J. (1974) Multi-infarct dementia. A cause of mental deterioration in the elderly. Lancet ii:207–210.

Hachinski, V.C. et al. (1975) Cerebral blood flow in dementia. Arch. Neurol. 32:632–637.

Hakim, A.M. and Mathieson, G. (1978) Basis of dementia in Parkinson's disease. Lancet ii:729.

Hall, P. (1966) Clinical aspects of moving house as a precipitant of psychiatric symptoms. J. Psychosom. Res. 10:59–80.

Hall, P. (1974) Differential diagnosis and treatment of depression in the elderly. Gerontol. Clin. 16:1–3, 126–136.

Hare, M. (1978) Clinical check list for diagnosis of dementia. Br. Med. J. 2:266–267.

Harrow, M., Grinker, R.R., Silverstein, M.M., and Holzmann, P. (1978) Is the modern-day schizophrenic outcome still negative? Am. J. Psychiatry 135:1156–1162.

Heiser, J.F. and De Francisco, D. (1976) The treatment of pathological panic states with propranolol. Am. J. Psychiatry 133:1389–1394.

Heston, L.L. and Mastri, A.R. (1977) The genetics of Alzheimer's disease. Arch. Gen. Psychiatry 34:976–981.

Hildick-Smith, M. (1974) A typical journey to and from the day hospital. Gerontol. Clin. 16:263–269.

Hodkinson, H.M. (1972) Evaluation of a mental test score for assessment of mental impairment in the elderly. Age and Aging 1:233–238.

Hodkinson, H.M. (1976) Common Symptoms of Disease in the Elderly. Oxford, Blackwell.

Hollinder, M.H. and Goldin, M.L. (1978) Funeral mania. J. Nerv. Ment. Dis. 166:890–892.

Hunter, R.A., Dayan, A.D., and Wilson, J. (1972) Alzheimer's disease in one monozygotic twin. J. Neurol. Neurosurg. Psychiatry 35:707–710.

Irvine, R.E. (ed) (1974) Symposium on day care. Gerontol. Clin. Vol. 16, Nos. 5 and 6.

Jackson, G. J., Pierscianowski, T. A., Mahon, W., and Condon, J. (1976) Inappropriate antihypertensive therapy in the elderly. Lancet ii:1317—1318.

Jankovic, B. D., Jakulic, S., and Horvat, J. (1977) Cerebral atrophy, an immunological disorder? Lancet ii:219—220.

Jarvik, L. F. (1974) Mental function related to chromosome findings in the aged. Series 274. Amsterdam, Excerpta Medica, pp. 851—855.

Jarvik, L. F., Altschuler, K. Z., Kato, T., and Blumner, B. (1971) Organic brain syndrome and chromosome loss in aged twins. Dis. Nerv. Syst. 32:159—170.

Johnstone, E. C. and Marsh, W. (1973) Acetylator status and response to phenelzine in depressed patients. Lancet i:567—570.

Judge, T. G., Urquhart, A., and Blakemore, C. B. (1973) Cyclandelate and mental functions. Age and Aging 2:171—124.

Kahlbaum, K. L. (1874) Die Katatonie. Berlin, Kirschwald.

Kahn, R. L., Pollack, M., and Goldfarb, A. I. (1961) Factors relative to individual differences in mental states of the institutionalised aged. In Hock, P. H. and Zubin, J. Psychopathology of Aging. New York, Grune and Stratton.

Kaplitz, S. E. (1975) Withdrawn, apathetic geriatric patients responsive to methylphenidate. J. Am. Geriatr. Soc. 23:271—276.

Karacan, I. Advances in the diagnosis of erectile impotence. Med. Asp. Hum. Sexual. 12:85, 1978.

Kay, D. W. K., Bergmann, K., Foster, E. M., and Garside, R. F (1966) A four year follow up of a random sample of old people seen originally in their own homes. In Proc. IV World Congr. Psychiatry. Madrid and Amsterdam, Excerpta Medica.

Klein, D. F. (1964) Delineation of two drug-responsive anxiety syndromes. Psychopharmacologic 5:397—408.

Kurland, M. L. (1979) Organic brain syndrome with propranolol. N. Engl. J. Med. 300:366.

Kurucz, J., Feldman, G., and Werner, W. (1979) Prosopo-affective agnosia associated with chronic brain syndrome. J. Am. Geriatr. Soc. 27:91—95.

Lassen, N. A., Ingvar, D. H., Skinhøj, E. (1978) Brain function and blood flow. Sci. Am. 239:62—71.

Legros, J.J. et al. (1978) Influence of vasopressin on learning and memory. Lancet i:41—42.

Lehmann, H. L. and Ban, T. A. (1975) In Gershon, S. and Raskin, A. Genesis and treatment of psychological disorders in the elderly. New York, Raven Press pp. 179—202.

Lewis, N. D. C. and Piotrowski, Z. A. (1954) Clinical diagnosis of manic depressive psychosis. In Hock, P. and Zubin, J. Depression. New York, Grune and Stratton.

Linn, L. (1975) In Freedman, A. M., Kaplan, H. I., and Sadock, B. J. Comprehensive Textbook of Psychiatry. Vol. 1. Baltimore, Williams and Wilkins, p. 813.

Liston, E. H. (1977) Occult presenile dementia. J. Nerv. Ment. Dis. 164:263—267.

Luisada, A. A. and Jacobs, R. (1969) Action of a vasodilator on the circulation of the skull and brain. Vasc. Dis. 3:3.

Maas, J. W. (1975) Biogenic amines and depression. Arch. Gen. Psychiatry 32:1357—1361.

McDermott, J. R., Smith, A. I., Igbal, K., and Wisniewski, H. M. (1977) Aluminum and Alzheimer's disease. Lancet ii:710—711.

Mann, A. H. (1973) Cortical atrophy and air encephalography: a clinical and radiological study. Psychol. Med. 3:374—378.

Manschreck, T. C. and Petri, M. (1978) The paranoid syndrome. Lancet ii:251−253.

Marsden, C. D. (1978) The diagnosis of dementia. *In* Isaacs, A. D. and Post, F. Studies in Geriatric Psychiatry. Chichester, John Wiley.

Martin, W. E., Loewenson, R. B., Resch, J. A., and Baker, A. B. (1973) Parkinson's disease: Clinical analysis of 100 patients. Neurol. (Minneap.) 23:783−790.

Mayeux, R. (1979) Sexual intercourse and transient global amnesia. N. Engl. J. Med. 300:864.

Milton, G. W. (1973) Self-willed death, or the bone-pointing syndrome. Lancet i:1435−1436.

Nausieda, P. A. and Sherman, I. C. (1979) Long-term prognosis in transient global amnesia. J.A.M.A. 241:392−393.

O'Brien, M. D. and Veall, N. (1966) Effects of cyclandelate on cerebral cortex perfusion rates in cerebrovascular disease. Lancet ii:729.

Oliveros, J.C. et al. (1978) Vasopressin in amnesia. Lancet i:42.

Olsson, J. E., Muller, R., and Berneli, S. (1976) Long term anticoagulant therapy for TIAs and minor strokes with minimum residua. Stroke 7:444−451.

Perry, E. K., Perry, R. H., and Tomlinson, B. E. (1977) Dietary lecithin supplements in dementia of Alzheimer type? Lancet ii:242−243.

Philips, M. J. and Felix, D. (1976) Specific angiotensin II receptive neurones in the cat subfornical organ. Brain Res. 109:531−540.

Pomerance, A. (1972) Cardiac pathology in the aged. Mod. Geriatr. 2:140−145.

Ponto, L. B., Perry, P. J., Liskow, B. I., and Seaba, H. H. (1977) Drug therapy reviews: Tricyclic antidepressant and MAOI combination therapy. Am. J. Hosp. Pharm. 34:954−961.

Pope, H. G. and Lipinski, J. F. (1978) Diagnosis in schizophrenia and manic depressive illness. Arch. Gen. Psychiatry 35:811−828.

Post, F. (1968) The factor of aging in affective illness. *In* Oppen, A. and Walk, A. Recent developments in affective disorders. Br. J. Psychiatry, Special Publication 2.

Post, F. (1978) The functional psychoses. *In* Isaacs, A. D. and Post, F. Studies in Geriatric Psychiatry. Chichester, John Wiley.

Prinsley, D. M. (1978) The geriatric physician's role in assessment and management. *In* Isaacs, A. D. and Post, F. Studies in Geriatric Psychiatry. Chichester, John Wiley, pp. 211−218.

Rao, D. B., Georgiev, E. L., Paul, P. D., and Guzman, A. B. (1977) Cyclandelate in the treatment of senile mental changes: A double-blind evaluation. J. Am. Geriatr. Soc. 25:548−551.

Raskin, A. (1972) Adverse reactions to phenalzine—results of a nine hospital study. J. Clin. Pharmacol. 12:22−25.

Raskin, D. E. (1977) Akathisia—a side effect to be remembered. Am. J. Psychiatry 129:345−347.

Rickarby, G. A. (1977) Four cases of mania with bereavement. J. Nerv. Ment. Dis. 165:255−262.

Robinson, D. S., and Nies, A., Ravaris, C. L., Ives, J. O., and Bartlett, D. (1978) Clinical pharmacology of phenelzine. Arch. Gen. Psychiatry 35:629−635.

Roth, M. (1971) Classification and aetiology in mental disorders of old age. *In* Kay, D. W. K. and Walk, A. Recent Developments in Psychogeriatrics, Br. J. Psychiatry. Special Publication 6:1−8.

Roth, M. and Morrissey, J. D. (1952) Problems of diagnosis and classification of mental disorders in old age. J. Ment. Sci. 98:66−80.

Salkind, M. R. (1970) The use of sustained-release lithium carbonate in general practice. J. R. Coll. Gen. Pract. 20:13–21.

Salzman, C. and Shader, R. I. (1975) Psychopharmacology in the aged. J. Geriatr. Psychiatry 7:165–184.

Sathanathan, G. L. and Gershon, S. (1975) In Gershon, S. and Raskin, A. Genesis and treatment of psychological disorders in the elderly. New York, Raven Press, pp. 155–168.

Saul, L. J. (1965) Dream scintillations. Psychosom. Med. 27:286–290.

Scheibel, M. E. and Scheibel, A. B. Structural changes in the aging brain. In Brody, A., Harman, D., and Ordy, J. M. Clinical, Morphologic and Neurochemical Aspects in the Aging C.N.S. New York, Raven Press.

Schildkraut, J. J., Keeler, B. A., Papousek, M., et al. (1973) MHPG excretion in depressive disorders. Relation to clinical subtypes and desynchronised sleep. Science 18:762–764.

Schneider, K. (1959) Clinical Psychopathology. (Hamilton, M. W. trans.). New York, Grune and Stratton.

Seltzer, B. and Sherwin, I. (1978) Organic brain syndromes: An empirical study and critical review. Am. J. Psychiatry 124:13–21.

Shader, R. I., Harmatz, J. S., and Salzman, C. (1974) A new scale for clinical assessment in geriatric populations—Sandoz Clinical Assessment Geriatric (SCAG). J. Am. Geriatr. Soc. 22.107–113.

Shuckit, M., Robins, E., and Feighner, J. (1971) Tricyclic antidepressants and monoamine oxidase inhibitors: Combination therapy in the treatment of depression. Arch. Gen. Psychiatry 24:509–514.

Signoret, J. L., Whiteley, A., and Lhermitte, F. (1978) Influence of choline on amnesia in early Alzheimer's disease. Lancet ii:837.

Sjogren, T., Sjogren, H., and Lundgren, A. G. H. (1963) Morbus Alzheimer and morbus Pick: A genetic, clinical and neuroanatomic study. Acta Psychiatr. Scand. (Suppl.) 82.

Solomon, F., White, C. C., Parron, D. L., and Mendelsohn, W. B. Sleeping pills, insomnia and medical practice. N. Engl. J. Med. 300:803–808.

Stotsky, B. A. (1975) In Gershon, S. and Raskin, A. Aging 2: Genesis and Treatment of Psychologic Disorders in the Elderly. New York, Raven Press, pp. 252–253.

Strouthidis, T. M. (1974) Medical requirements of a day hospital. Gerontol. Clin. 16:241–247.

Summers, W. K. and Reich, T. C. (1979) Delirium after cataract surgery: Review and two cases. Am. J. Psychiatry 136:386–391.

Tarter, R. E. (1975) Psychological deficit in chronic alcoholics: A review. Int. J. Addict. 10:327–368.

Thomson, I. (1977) Integration of psychiatric assessment for the elderly. Lancet ii:239–240.

Tyrer, P. (1976) Towards rational therapy with monoamine oxidase inhibitors. Br. J. Psychiatry 128:354–360.

Van Boxell, P., Bridges, P. K., Bartlett, J. R., and Trauer, T. (1978) Size of cerebral ventricles in 66 psychiatric patients. Br. J. Psychiatry 133:500–506.

Van Putten, T. (1975) The many faces of akathisia. Compr. Psychiatry 16:43–47.

Victor, M., Adams, R. D., and Collins, G. H. (1971) The Wernicke–Korsakoff syndrome. Philadelphia, Davis.

Walsh, A. C. and Walsh, B. H. (1974) Presenile dementia—further experience with an anticoagulant-psychotherapy regimen. J. Am. Geriatr. Soc. 22:467–472.

Walsh, A. C. and Lukas, E. (1974) Alcoholic brain damage: Anticoagulant therapy. J. Am. Geriatr. Soc. 22:555—556.

Walsh, A. C., Walsh, B. H., and Melaney, C. (1978) Senile-presenile dementia: Follow-up data on an effective psychotherapy-anticoagulant regimen. J. Am. Geriatr. Soc. 26:467—470.

Wartenburg, R. (1952) Head-dropping test. Br. Med. J. 1:687—689.

Watson, C. G. and Thomas, R. W. (1968) MMPI profiles of brain-damaged and schizophrenic patients. Percept. Mot. Skills 27:567—573.

Weiss, J. M. A. (1973) The natural history of antisocial attitudes. J. Geriatr. Psychiatry 6:236—242.

Wells, C. E. (1978) Chronic brain disease, an overview. Am. J. Psychiatry 135:1—12.

Wilson, L. A. and Brass, W. (1973) Brief assessment of the mental state in geriatric domiciliary practise. Age and Aging 2:92—101.

Wisniewski, H. M., Terry, R. D., and Hirano, A. (1970) Neurofibrillary pathology. J. Neuropathol. Exp. Neurol. 29:163—176.

Wurtman, J. R., Hirsch, M. J., and Growdon, J. H. (1977) Lecithin consumption raises serum-free-choline levels. Lancet ii:68.

Yesavage, J. A., Hollister, L. E., and Burian, E. (1979a) Dihydroergotoxine: 6 mg versus 3 mg dosage in the treatment of senile dementia. J. Am. Geriatr. Soc. 27:80—82.

Yesavage, J. A., Tinklenberg, J. R., Hollister, L. E., and Berger, P. (1979b) Vasodilators in senile dementias. Arch. Gen. Psychiatry 36:220—223.

Yorkston, N. J., Gruzelier, J. H., Zaki, S. A., Hollander, D., Pitcher, D. R., and Sergeant, H. G. S. (1977) Propranolol as an adjunct to the treatment of schizophrenia. Lancet ii:575—578.

INDEX

N

Neurochemistry
    and Alzheimerism, 47, 48
    and depression, 23–24, 26
    and schizophrenia, 33
Neurosis, 26, 69–70, 71
Neurotic depression, 26
Nocturnal confusion, 74, 76
"Nursing home dementia," 8–9
Nursing observation scale, 58

O

Opiates, 76
Organic dementing processes, 3, 36,
    41–57

P

Panic, 6–7
Paraldehyde, 4
Paranoia, 5, 14, 36–39
Parkinsonism, 2, 14, 45–46, 47, 48
Phenothiazines, 4, 5, 30, 34, 36, 37, 75
Physical disease. See also Somatization
    and mental symptoms, 12
    presentation of, 1
Physician
    attitudes of, 19, 59, 63–65
    education of, for geriatrics, 92, 94–97
    family, 87–88
    role of, 1
    and understanding of aging, 63–65
Pick's dementia, 41
Propranolol, 7, 35–36
Pseudodementia, 8–9, 12, 42
Psychiatry, geriatric
    clientele of, 2
    and the law, 81–84
Psychogeriatric assessment center, 88,
    89–91
"Psychopathic personalities," 79
Psychoses, major, 20–41. See also
    specific type
Psychotherapy, 6, 16, 26, 28, 63–73

R

Raven block tests, 62
Raven progressive matrices, 58
Reactive depression, 4

Rehabilitation, 81
REM rebound, 75
Roles, 69
Rorschach inkblots, 58–59

S

Sandoz Geriatric Assessment Scale, 58
Schizoaffective illness, 33, 34
Schizophrenia, 3, 32–39
    first-rank symptoms of, 5, 33, 34, 35,
        39
    paranoid, 39
Self-value, sources of, 63, 65, 66, 68
"Senility," 1, 8, 9, 10–19
    and abnormal behavior, 14–15
    definition of, 10
    and family's role, 17–18
    investigation of, 15–17
    and memory loss, 14
    as mental symptom, 12–13
    presentation of, 11–12
    as role, 77
    and weakness, 13–14
Sensory deficits, 5
Sex counseling, 85, 90
Sexuality, 38, 84–86, 90
Sleep patterns, 7, 14, 74–77
Slowing, 18
Sodium depletion, 14
Somatization, 4, 21, 66
Sulfinpyrazone, 51–52
Suicide, 4, 27, 28, 31
Syndrome of inappropriate antidiuretic
    hormone secretion (SIADH), 14

T

Tests, mental. See Mental tests
Thiamine, 53
Thiothixenes, 35
Thyroid disorders, 13
Thyroid extract, 32
Tomographic scanning, 43–44
Transference, 6
Tricyclic antidepressants, 4, 23, 24, 25,
    26, 27, 28, 29–30, 35
L-tryptophan, 32

V

Vasodilators, 42, 52–53, 57